GAS
MAN

COLIN BLACK

GAS MAN

Observations of an Anaesthetist

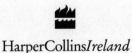

HarperCollins*Ireland*

HarperCollins*Publishers*
1 London Bridge Street
London SE1 9GF

www.harpercollins.co.uk

HarperCollins*Ireland*
1st Floor, Watermarque Building, Ringsend Road
Dublin 4, Ireland

First published by HarperCollins*Ireland* 2021

3 5 7 9 10 8 6 4 2

A catalogue record of this book is
available from the British Library

ISBN 978-0-00-847014-2

Printed and bound in the UK using 100%
renewable electricity at CPI Group (UK) Ltd

ABOUT THE AUTHOR

Dr Colin Black was born in Derry City but has lived in Dublin since the age of 3, so has long since traded his calming northwestern lilt for a posh South Dublin accent. Colin is a Consultant Paediatric Anaesthesiologist with a special interest in anaesthesia for congenital heart disease, and has worked in hospitals across Ireland, following a period of 'finding himself' in Australia. His anaesthesia finishing school was the esteemed Great Ormond Street Hospital for Children in central London.

Now based at Children's Health Ireland at Crumlin, Colin lives in Dublin with his wife, who also happens to be a surgeon, and their young daughter, whom they hope does not become a doctor too.

For the little chicken.
And the bigger chicken.

CONTENTS

AUTHOR'S NOTE

To protect the identity of patients, their parents and colleagues, I have altered names and clinical details throughout this book. I encounter many patients with similar clinical problems, therefore any resemblance is coincidental. Some colleagues will, of course, easily decipher that I am making reference to them. I have sought their permission to publish any glaringly obvious identifying details. Hopefully everyone else will still have a cup of mediocre hospital tea with me. Despite these alterations, this is not a work of fiction and all of the anecdotes, stories and musings are true and were composed in a one-year period.

OBSERVATION

An Introduction

Definition: Observation is the subtle art of shutting up, putting away the phone and simply paying attention every now and again.

Quiet observation of patients was (and one could argue still is) the cornerstone of medicine. If you look back at historical artwork portraying doctors, what do you see? There is no scalpel, no blood pressure cuff, no oxygen, often not even a nurse to assist. There is a pensive man – always a man – sitting in a candlelit room. Parents or family of the suffering patient look on in fear, a wash of angst across their faces. The patient lies in bed, sweating, panting, with a ghastly sense of doom emanating from their eyes. The doctor watches, hand on chin. He looks closer. He observes the pattern of breathing, the number of breaths, the look in the patient's eyes. He palpates the pulse and feels how it changes over time. He observes the colour of the skin change as the last lease of life drains from the patient. A sigh.

Descriptions like the scene above occurred in the Victorian era, just before the cusp of modern medicine. We now have many tools to aid our observations and make accurate diagnoses. The skill of observation is waning, with doctors ever more dependent on machines to do the work for us. Anaesthetists spend all day, every day, making observations. We are hyperaware of our surroundings. We continuously observe, as our unconscious patients lack the capacity to tell us when things are wrong. We look for patterns in everything: the vital signs, the mechanics of the ventilator, the body language of the surgeon, the change of atmosphere in the room. Just like doctors of old, the more you observe, the more patterns you will see and the quicker you can intervene when something isn't right.

Despite this sombre introduction, I wouldn't want you to think all anaesthetists sit by candlelight with a pipe hanging from their bottom lip before coming to the conclusion that what the patient needs are a few leeches to the anus. When the patterns are normal and the anaesthetic is going well, I find myself observing everything else that goes on in the operating theatre: how staff interact, how the hospital runs or how patients experience a new and intimidating environment. What you can learn from sitting quietly and making observations is limitless.

This book is full of my clinical and not-so-clinical observations from the journey to becoming a consultant anaesthetist and my first year on the job.

PART 1

How to Become an Anaesthetist

Medicine

I didn't always want to be a doctor. It's not the family business; there are no doctors in my family. I surprised myself and my parents with my Leaving Certificate points haul, beating my parents' predictions by 80 and 85 points respectively.[1] 'How did *you* get *those* points, Colin?' asked my form teacher. *I literally have no idea.* So, I headed into University College Dublin (UCD) as a physiotherapy student, determined to become part of the set-up at a Premier League football club. Picking up Dennis Bergkamp from the pitch, dinner parties with Patrick Vieira, charades with Tony Adams, playing golf with Thierry Henry. That was the job I wanted. Unbeknownst to me, the role of a physiotherapist consists of a lot more than picking up overpaid prima donnas from a football pitch.

---

1 They even made a bet with each other. The Leaving Cert (the Irish equivalent to the A-levels if you're from the UK) was scored out of 600 when I sat it, with entry to medicine requiring at least 530 points but often many more.

It was during one practical session in which we learned how to vigorously expel sputum from the murky depths of a patient's lungs, or perhaps another on how to help to stabilise the pelvic floor during pregnancy, that I decided that this career wasn't for me. I barely passed the first practical exam at Christmas. But what I had discovered was the subject of physiology: how the body works. The only way for me to pursue this further was by studying medicine. After one year of life as an unenthusiastic physiotherapy student, I made the switch, scraping my way into medicine. I was yet again entirely naïve as to what sort of life I was embarking on.

Our system for entry into university is not a good one. In the minority of cases, a teenager has a burning desire to be a doctor/ police officer/trapeze artist, and always has done. The fact is, though, that the majority of teenagers haven't the faintest idea what they want to do. How can you when you've spent most of the last five years trying to become a professional footballer or an Instagram influencer? Medicine is a very interpersonal and communication-heavy vocation. Social skills and emotional intelligence are almost half the job. There are some doctors I know who would be best placed in a back office, well away from any human interaction, for the sake of both parties.[2] There are many doctors who found their way into the profession by simply retaining and regurgitating facts on one sunny day in June better than the other candidates.

Studying medicine is hard. It's not that the concepts are exceedingly difficult or abstract at undergraduate level, it's the immense size of the syllabus. You literally learn everything about the human body. We learned the syllabus in blocks, from the ground up. First, anatomy, physiology and biochemistry – the basic sciences of medicine.

---

2 Thankfully, since I sat the Leaving Cert, there have been drastic changes to the entry requirements for medicine. Less, 'I'll do medicine just because I have the points.' A more complicated entry process now includes an aptitude test which aims to recruit people who want to study for the right reasons. Would I get into medicine if I applied now? I have no idea.

For example, the renal system. Renal anatomy: what are the anatomical relations of the kidney in the abdomen, label the anatomical features of the kidney, what is the blood supply, what is the nervous supply, what is the histological appearance of the kidney? Exam question: *Describe the anatomical features of the urinary system with emphasis on blood and nervous supply.* Next, renal physiology: what are the functions of the kidney, how does it perform these duties, where are some of the therapeutic drug targets within the kidney? *Explain the role of the renal system in arterial blood pressure regulation.* Then, renal biochemistry: what cellular mechanisms are involved in these processes, how does it affect your electrolyte homeostasis and fluid balance? *Draw and label the structure of the nephron and emphasise mechanisms used to control sodium resorption.*

Next we move on to when things go wrong. We learn how to diagnose and how to treat various ailments: pathology and pharmacology. Staying with the kidneys, renal pathology: cancer, vasculitides, glomerulonephritides, drug injuries, auto-immune disease, congenital abnormalities.[3] *Compare and contrast nephrotic and nephritic syndromes.* Then, renal pharmacology: what drugs affect the function of the kidney, what biochemical receptors do they target, how do they work, what are the desired effects, what are the side effects? *Classify diuretic medication with emphasis on the mechanism of action within the nephron.* This process is repeated for every single organ system in the body. Breathe, but don't rest; you're only half-way through. That's just the 'pre-clinical' years.

Next, the 'clinical' years, covering rotations in medicine, surgery, obstetrics, paediatrics and psychiatry begin. Hundreds of medical students are released into the hospital system to spend the next two and a half years trying to make sense of it all. Heads bursting with new words, speaking in tongues. *Pneumothorax, Wegener's*

---

3 Congenital means 'present from birth'.

granulomatosis, Virchow's triad, carbamazepine, schistosomiasis.
White coats bleached and pressed by proud mothers. Some cheeky
bastards even put on a stethoscope, but it's far too soon for that.[4]
Those who prematurely bear the weight of the stethoscope across
their shoulders will shrink in confidence after a dressing-down or
two from a real doctor, and quickly stuff the offending guess-o-
scopes back into their pockets. We nervously escort each other
around the wards, the blind leading the blind, a bunch of lemmings
plunging over a cliff into the frosty sea, squealing inappropriate
diagnoses and irrelevant investigations. 'What investigation would
you like to perform for migraine?' *Em, a brain biopsy?*

At this point we begin to learn the core elements of being a
doctor: the skill of history-taking – asking the patient all the relevant questions about why they have come to see you – and clinical
examination, examining the patient for evidence of the disease
process you suspect to be the problem, based on the questions you
asked. We disperse and roam the wards. We are initially quiet as
mice, not wanting to get in anyone's way. But closer to exams, we
are more like bleating goats, head-butting our way onto crowded
wards.

On escaping from our cages, we start by relentlessly pestering the
nurses. 'Are there are any patients we could talk to or examine?'
The nurses pull out the patient list and point us in the direction of
beds 6 and 9.[5] Medical students are very discerning in whom they
choose to interview on the wards. *Hhhhmmmm.* We can be seen

---

4 Any medical student caught actually wearing a stethoscope by their
classmates will be mocked and jeered for having 'notions' about
themselves actually being mistaken for a real doctor. It should be hidden
well inside your pocket until you earn it.

5 It is a bad habit we have in hospitals where staff refer to actual real,
living human beings by their bed number or diagnosis. 'Bed 4 needs her
aspirin.' 'Where's the laparotomy from yesterday?' 'Does the kidney stone
need pain relief?'

coyly screwing our heads inside the wards, ogling the suggested patients. It is imperative you have a good gawk before committing. You shouldn't judge a book by its cover, but by God we judged all those books. Bed 6 appears to be asleep but wakens to start chatting animatedly to the fruit hamper left in by Annie from next door. Bed 9 just doesn't look like a good patient; you can't put your finger on it. This won't do. Medical students are picky. We go back to the source and ask for another recommendation. Interrupting the nurse twice is not acceptable: it's 3.10 p.m. and she has eight more patients to get to in the 2 p.m. medication round. We get the message to move on to another ward.

We saunter down to the adjacent ward and meet a classmate in the corridor:

'Any good histories? Any signs?'

This is a frequent question. A 'sign' is a positive finding on clinical examination such as a heart murmur or a lump in the abdomen or a hamster in the rectum. God help you if you are ever in a hospital as a patient with a 'good sign'. Be warned, it is not a good sign for you, as you will have a queue of medical students out the door asking you to expose your abdomen/boobs/genitalia. If you seem particularly comfortable with the students you'll almost certainly be asked to take part in the medical examinations as a live subject.

When a diligent medical student has been brave enough to take a full history and examine a patient, they will seek out a real doctor and ask if they can 'present' the case. Presenting a case is also a core skill, as you use this technique to talk to superiors and peers for the rest of your career. The idea is to summarise the reason a patient is in hospital and their relevant medical history, present the findings of your clinical examination and come up with a differential diagnosis (what *might* be wrong with the patient). You follow this with a list of tests you might request to confirm your suspicions, and offer some potential treatment plans. The key is to present only what is relevant. Novices at presenting a history will insist on telling the listener what size shoe Frank bought from TK Maxx last week as if it were a clue as to why he has been having explosive diarrhoea.

Presenting a case to a new intern is not daunting as they will be helpful and offer pointers on how to keep it succinct. Presenting a case to a registrar is scarier, as they will point out all your omissions and your shortcomings as a human being, then sigh as they realise that the break they had been looking forward to will now be spent straightening out medical students. But if you are presenting to a consultant, you better hope you put on a second pair of underpants that morning. They can be scathing and intimidating, but crucially they are training you to be accurate and precise, as this is what is necessary when you call a superior at 3 a.m. asking for advice.

I owe my medical degree to a professor of obstetrics and gynaecology. He scared the living daylights out of everyone. He detested tardiness and untidiness. He could see through a bullshitter with a passing glance. He remembered everyone. On our first day, 40 of us sat in the lecture theatre as he called the roll. With each response, he glared and imprinted each face into his vast mental catalogue of medical students. He forgot no one's name. Ever.

'Mr Black, you're on nights in the labour ward this week.'

What the …? Nights? I'm a student, I go drinking at night. I sleep for 11 hours a day.

'Yes, professor.'

We heard that he hovered around the halls at night wearing a black cape. But, if you managed to overcome your terror in his forbidding presence – and if you knew your stuff, he would pat you on the back and say well done. I have never studied so hard in my life. I wanted that pat on my back. I learned everything there is to know about pregnancy, the female menstrual cycle and where to find the clitoris. This was all to avoid his wrath. I didn't intend to do well, it was all an avoidance exercise, but I achieved first-class honours in my final obstetric exam. It might have been a first achieved through the modus of fear, but it showed me what I was capable of and what level of dedication was required to make it.

The last of the clinical years is the formative year. You follow the doctors around more, you rotate through different specialties, you go to the operating theatre for a close-up view of real surgery. You get a sense of what the job is really about, you start to think like a doctor and, hopefully, you get a feeling for what specialty interests you. All the exams from this point are largely clinical – meaning they are with a real patient. Although it's supposed to be where you can demonstrate your knowledge, it can be a frightful experience.

The crux of the clinical exam is the 'long case'. On exam day, an invigilator meets you at the entrance to the ward and, with a curt smile, gently guides you to a room on the ward. A curtain is drawn and you meet the gaze of the expectant patient in front of you. Suddenly, you are thrown in to the bedside with the briefest of introductions and 20 minutes later, on the button, the examiners all arrive. The examiners, all being consultants, naturally cut you off mid-sentence. You present the case, offering a differential diagnosis and how you might treat the patient. The ideal scenario is to have a medical patient when one of the examiners happens to be a surgeon, or vice-versa, a surgical patient when one of the examiners happens to be a physician. At least in this case, you can assume the surgeon isn't completely up to speed with the latest high-tech immunomodulating drugs used to treat chronic rheumatological problems, and thus won't be quizzing you on them. Not that you know anything about them either. The worst scenario is seeing the professor of medicine, with her head bursting with the latest research developments across the entire medical spectrum, walk in and you've been extracting information piecemeal from a suitably demented medical patient and thus have no clear information for your performance. After your limp presentation, there follows a barrage of questions. You attempt to duck and weave your way through the entry-level questions for a pass. You sweat and flounder your way through the honours questions. An almost deathly silence descends as you attempt to describe the histological appearance of Langerhans Cell Histiocytosis to a consultant haematologist for first-class honours. Your body starts to incinerate itself from the inside before, mercifully, they let your burning carcass rest inside that once-pristine white coat. Off to the pub to dissect the exam. *Am I a doctor yet?*

To a medical student used to spending almost an hour talking with a patient on the wards, 20 minutes to chat to a patient in an exam scenario is not much time at all. Often, these extended pre-exam practice chats are the result of being too polite to redirect an elderly pensioner back from his tales of life as a young whippersnapper climbing trees in Mullingar to the salient question of why he is in the hospital in the first place. Come exam time, politeness goes out the window. You have 20 minutes to extract all the information out of a poor patient who is being asked the same questions for the fourth time today.

'So, Mary, what brought you to the hospital?'

'I had a turn.'

'Ok, what do you mean by a turn?'

'I felt a funny thing.'

Suddenly it feels hot in the room.

'Can you be more specific, Mary?'

'Well, it's like when you know something is not quite right, you know?'

'Did you have pain?'

'Not really.'

A bead of sweat forms on your brow.

'Did you have trouble breathing?'

'No. Are you from Dublin or do you just go to college here?'

'I'm from Dublin, Mary. Did you vomit? Did you faint? Were you short of breath?'

'I went to UCD years ago. It used to be all fields around here you know.'

JesusfuckingChrist, Mary, answer the bloody question! The examiners will be here in 11 minutes and I haven't a fucking clue what's wrong with you!

Doctor

For me, choosing my medical subspecialty was a process of elimination. As I never knew I wanted to study medicine, I certainly had never given any thought to what type of doctor I wanted to be. My wife is a senior surgical trainee in urology. Her father is a surgeon. For as long as she can remember, she always wanted to be a surgeon. Many of my friends are general practitioners (GPs) and they have always wanted to follow that path to follow their parents. I started narrowing down a mental list in my final year of medicine based on what I felt to be valid reasoning. Surgery – too long to train, what if I'm just shit at it? Obstetrics – too high risk, don't want to be sued. GP – too much talking. Pathology – not enough talking. Radiology – too lonely, would spend too much money on coffee. Psychiatry – my beard is not strong enough. Internal medicine – too many endless ward rounds and overbooked clinics. My goal appeared to be a specialty with a moderate length of training, in which I wouldn't spend *all* my money on legal advice or coffee, or have to talk to patients either too much or too little, with instant gratification and no ward rounds. I had my intern year to ponder this conundrum.

The hospital hierarchy from the most junior position up is as follows: intern (also known as house officer, or your foundation year in the UK), senior house officer (SHO), registrar, specialist registrar (SpR), fellow (only in some hospitals), then, finally, consultant.[6] As an intern, although you are a bona fide doctor, you really have the role of administrative officer for your assigned team. It feels more like being a medical student with a folder and a list of patients rather than real clinical doctoring, certainly during daylight hours. The day job consisted of begging other specialties for consults, begging radiology for CT and MRI scans and begging the nurses to cut us some slack. *Please just do it! My consultant wants a CT scan, I don't know why. PLEASE.* We were sweaty beggars roaming the hospital with enough paper under our arms to start a decent forest fire. By the end of the day, we were expected to have followed up on results of various investigations and have all the information to hand for when your registrar or consultant embarked on a ward round. It is flat out, but mostly clerical work.

As an intern, you are 'on call' at night on the wards and thus have a bit more legitimate medical facetime with patients. However, there are several more senior doctors to call immediately if any patient is looking a little ropey. The majority of your calls from the nursing staff at night are still for mundane tasks such as charting pain relief or siting a new intravenous (IV) cannula. The IV cannula – the gateway to drug administration, the bane of the life of an intern. Why is something so simple and inane more troubling than

---

6 I use registrar and specialist registrar interchangeably throughout the book. Technically speaking, if you're interested, the specialist registrar is one who is on an officially recognised training scheme administered by the college of their relevant specialty. E.g. the surgical SpR has gained entry onto the higher training scheme administered by the College of Surgeons, etc. Some skip the 'registrar' phase and go straight to specialist registrar. Some registrars are more experienced than specialist registrars. If you were a registrar in one specialty then changed to another, you'll probably be demoted to SHO. Fellows are those doing extra, super-specialised work after completing life as a specialist registrar and before taking up a consultant post. But not all consultant posts require you to have worked as a fellow. Confused? Excellent. I'll just refer to anyone more senior than an SHO, but more junior than a consultant, as being a 'registrar'. But I'll probably forget I made this promise in a few pages.

singlehandedly cracking the human genome for the fresh-faced intern? The perhaps shocking truth is that medical graduates do not have the faintest idea how to perform many of the elementary tasks one associates with being in the hospital (IV cannulas, urinary catheters, suturing of wounds). You learn and practise on real subjects, as an intern.

Let me give you an example. An arterial blood gas (ABG) is a sample of blood taken from an artery, usually performed if someone is looking fairly peaky, as it gives you heaps of very valuable information. It can tell you in mere minutes the pH of the blood, the blood oxygen and carbon dioxide levels, the haemoglobin, several important serum electrolytes (e.g. sodium, potassium) and the lactate level (a measure of anaerobic metabolism – not what you want). These are all fairly non-specific measures in that they tell you what is wrong, not why. You still need to use your brain somewhat. But if any of the measures are grossly abnormal, you'll need to take action soon to prevent further deterioration. Having an ABG sample taken hurts, but a registrar could take a sample with their eyes closed with one little poke in a second or two. Even after months as an intern, one former colleague of mine had such trouble with it, he would advise patients that the procedure would involve 'five or six little pokes in the wrist, and take about 15 minutes'. If he managed to successfully obtain the blood sample in only three or four attempts in half the time, the patient would be delighted. Medicine is all about managing expectations, I learned.

Interns wade through a lot of shite at night and over the weekends. Some patients decide that 3 a.m. is an appropriate time to ask for a doctor to discuss the minor ailment that they have been nursing for the last 15 years. 'I first noticed my ears getting blocked with wax after a holiday in Benidorm in 1986.' Frequently there are bizarre calls from the wards – review itchy eyebrow, patient found sitting on floor – please review, chart sleeping tablet for patient who is already asleep, swollen penis – please review. The intern who reviewed the swollen penis one night threw back the bed sheets to reveal a very impressive member indeed. He looked at the patient who grinned back and said, 'I call him Big Tom.' He reported back to the nurses that, yes, the man did indeed have a monstrous penis and thanked them for waking him from his precious hour of slumber to view it.

The day job was occasionally more interesting. As the cardiology intern, I had to supervise the exercise stress tests. This is a common test for patients who are suspected of having coronary artery disease. They are put to work on a treadmill, attached to a blood pressure and electrocardiogram (ECG) monitor, in order to see if they have any suspicious changes on their ECG trace while they exercise.[7] The test is stopped if a patient experiences chest pain or if there are ECG changes. Normally, the test doesn't last too long and supervising seemed a bit unnecessary to me. On my second day, a burly 39-year-old man arrived to be stress tested. Coronary artery disease in your thirties is highly unlikely so I expected this to be smooth running. As he pushed himself on the treadmill, his breathing got heavier. He started sweating but insisted that we let him continue; he was fine. There were no changes on his ECG, so we let him press on. More sweat, more panting. Then all of a sudden … *crash*. All 22 stone of him came crashing onto the safety rails of the treadmill. He was unconscious, suspended with one arm each trapped on a rail either side of the moving treadmill floor, with his feet being dragged along below. Our heads snapped to read the monitor: ventricular fibrillation, a cardiac arrest. I slammed the emergency stop button on the treadmill as the cardiac physiologist put out the call to the cardiac arrest team. As any parent will tell you, moving a sleeping child is a lot harder than it looks; moving

---

7 ECG is EKG in America because of course the correct spelling is cardiac with a k.

unconscious adult patients is like heaving a flaccid meat sack and it proved to be tough task for my 11-stone frame, assisted by a waif of a cardiac physiologist. But we managed to wrestle him to the floor of the stress room and started cardiopulmonary resuscitation (CPR). When the next person arrived, we had enough people to retrieve the defibrillator and shock him back to life. He had lost control of his bladder, as often happens, during the arrest and I was dripping in piss. He woke up quite quickly, a bit muddled, but not in bad shape. We had our answer anyway: he certainly had coronary artery disease, and went for coronary artery bypass surgery in the following days.

'Does this happen regularly'? I asked the consultant cardiologist, fearful that this was a weekly occurrence, unsure I could handle the stress of this on a regular basis.

'Not in at least ten years, but at least we got our answer. Well done,' was the reply.

So, intern year was *mostly* clerical work.

The cardiac arrest bleep might alarm for someone in a life-threatening emergency, at any time of the day. The arrest team consisted of designated interns, SHOs and registrars who were covering the wards. But it also includes an anaesthetist.[8] I had only come across the elusive anaesthetist briefly as a medical student. The whole specialty seemed strange to medical students. Who are these people who ghost in and out of the hospital? They didn't look like the stereotypical doctor. They had no defining features. No formal clothing, no stethoscopes, no folder full of paper. In the standard-issue theatre scrubs they could have been anyone. But I soon noticed that when an anaesthetist arrived during a dire emergency, everyone else seemed to relax. You heard them whisper,

---

8 I'm going to use the term 'anaesthetist' throughout this book, despite the fact that we are now technically 'anaesthesiologists' in Ireland, just like in North America. 'Anaesthetist' is still the most used title in Ireland and the UK.

'Thank God the anaesthetist is here.' Who were these ethereal beings who emanated Buddha-like tranquillity in the face of mass hysteria?

All I remembered from my one-week rotation in the operating theatre as a student was how god-awfully dull being an anaesthetist looked. Twiddle a few knobs on a machine, get grief from the surgeon and occasionally push some drugs through an IV cannula the size of a hosepipe. I genuinely felt it looked to be by far the shittiest medical job in the hospital.[9] I couldn't fathom why anyone would submit themselves to a life of such mind-numbing torture.

But it was only as an intern that I became taken by the calming effect of the anaesthetists in these scenarios. I was interested. They breezed in, made a rapid assessment, took quick action, calmed everyone down, intubated the patient with effortless flair, cannulated when no one else could and whisked the patient off to the intensive care unit (ICU) or theatre, all in the blink of an eye. At one point, my co-intern and I witnessed an anaesthetist ventilating a patient with one hand, talking to the ICU with a phone stuck under his cheek, moving the patient's bed down the corridor with his legs and I swear he was putting a nurse's phone number in his mobile phone with his free hand. We called them the 'shit-cool bastards'.

By the middle of my intern year I had decided by process of elimination that I wanted to be a cardiologist, an anaesthetist or an emergency doctor. They all seemed to fit my criteria. I had also decided at this point to move to Australia at the end of intern year. I felt that working in an emergency department (ED) in a hospital in Sydney's Northern Beaches would help me to make this career choice.

---

9 Except for proctology (sorry I couldn't resist).

Emergency Doctor

An ED is a fantastic place to work, and all doctors should be required to experience it for a period of time. It is both tremendously challenging and utterly hilarious. My skills in history-taking and performing a clinical exam were now at the required standard, and I had the whole thing down to a five-minute routine, the two aspects done simultaneously. Now I was also responsible for making actual clinical decisions about the treatment a patient needed (if any), and whether they needed to be admitted to hospital. I learned new skills, like moulding plaster casts, reading trauma x-rays and closing open wounds with sutures or glue. It wasn't always straightforward as I discovered when I glued my rubber glove to a six-year-old's head when attempting to close a wound. The shrill of the poor child as I attempted to remove it forced me to think outside the box. I severed the matted finger of the glove with scissors and sent him home with a single rubber finger attached to his head. It would fall off with the glue in a couple of days, I told his mum, happens all the time. She giggled – the poor boy did not – and took a photo.

My finest moment in the ED came as I steadied an elderly gentleman who was lying on his left side on a trolley in a private sideroom. He had severe back pain and I was planning on ruling out some serious pathology. I had my left hand on his right hip, which was ceiling-side up. I slid my right index finger up into his rectum[10] to check his anus was functioning satisfactorily (this is a legitimate examination in case you were thinking of reporting me); I gave clear instructions to 'squeeze my finger'. Nothing happened and there was some confused mumbling. Maybe it was my accent. The Australian nurse piped up, 'Suuuuhhhh, can you sqww-eeze 'is fingah?' Bemused, our elderly friend reached his left hand around

---

10 Sorry, I went from 0 to 100 mph with this story.

to his right hip and gently tugged on the index finger of my steadying hand. I didn't think I had to be quite so specific as to what finger I was referring to when one has been inserted into the rectum.[11] I tried to maintain my composure as the nurse assisting me appeared to be suppressing a laughter-induced seizure.

Yet again, though, even in the ED, with highly trained emergency doctors, the anaesthetist would be called in when things got serious in the resuscitation room. If a patient was critically unwell for any reason, the anaesthetist would be summoned to intubate the patient (or supervise the ED staff doing so) or place invasive monitoring lines. He or she would also need to make clinical decisions about the patient's treatment pathway; specifically, whether they needed to go immediately to theatre for surgery or to the ICU. What most people don't realise is that anaesthetists are trained both in anaesthesia and intensive care medicine. The vast majority of ICU physicians (intensivists) are trained anaesthetists. Anaesthesia, therefore, ticked all the boxes for me: emergency situations when you think on your feet; a specialty rich in basic sciences like physiology and pharmacology; many advanced procedural skills such as siting epidural catheters; and what was very appealing to me, having skills that no other doctors possess. They seemed to be the go-to doctors when patients are at their worst. I decided that emergency medicine wasn't for me, and I didn't have the heart – pardon the pun – to go through general internal medical training to become a cardiologist. So, after a year in Australia, it was back to Ireland to commence my six years of training to become an anaesthetist.

11 For the doctor reading who is concerned that if he didn't feel my finger tickling his anus, he therefore must have had cauda equina syndrome, you're wrong. Once he figured out which finger I was referring to, his anus nearly severed it, such was the vigour of his efforts.

Anaesthetist

I keep referring to the 'anaesthetist', but in Ireland, since 2018, we have become Americanised as 'anaesthesiologists'. I fear the change of name may be to gain some sort of legitimacy amongst the general public. I was once asked by a patient, as I prepared to anaesthetise him, if I had to go to do a night course to become an anaesthetist. Anaesthesia is just a bit beyond the scope of a six-week night course, and his question underlined how little people understand about anaesthesia and what an anaesthetist actually does.

Many people don't realise that we are, in fact, highly trained doctors who go through at least six years of postgraduate subspecialty training. But this doesn't bother me in the slightest. The days of the doctor being revered as the community soothsayer are gone. Patients are now empowered to take control of their care. The medic has become almost like a counsellor for a patient who is free to make fully informed choices regarding their health. We lay it on the table, you decide. If someone thinks my real job is playing bass in a U2 tribute band and I just do the anaesthesia gig on the side for a bit of extra cash, so be it, provided they understand and agree to the care I am about to impart on them or their child.

Another misunderstanding of the role of the anaesthetist is that we simply inject a medicine that sends you off to la-la land before we pack up our things and head to our offices to drink coffee and read the paper. While it may be true that we like our coffee, rest assured, we are with you the entire time you are in the operating theatre. We do your breathing for you, we supply your oxygen for you, we hydrate you, we supply your pain relief, we make sure you don't get cold, we monitor for changes in your condition based on what the surgeon is doing, we keep your sugar levels normal, we give blood if you are bleeding, we make sure you don't remember anything, we ensure you feel nothing, we protect you, we look after you. If we were simply to inject you with medication to induce anaesthesia and then promptly leave the operating room, there is a good chance you would die.[12] We need to be there all the time.

If I prepare well for a case, then I may well be sitting down appearing to do very little, but this is the aim. If I have managed to thoroughly assess a patient pre-operatively, planned for the requirements of not only the surgeon but the intra-operative requirements of the patient and contingency-planned for any potential complications, then what I get as a result is a patient who is completely clinically stable. They have normal oxygen levels, normal blood pressure, normal heart rate, normal temperature, no (or very little) pain and absolutely no recollection of anything. A chaotic anaesthetist unsettles everyone else in the operating theatre as we are the ones who are entirely responsible for the patient's safety. The more preparation, the less chaos. Chaos is distracting for the surgeon who needs to be focused to perform the operation successfully. If I get everything just right in this balancing act from the very start, I can then be completely focused on watching for any complicating events.

A huge amount of training as an anaesthetist is learning what to do when the unexpected happens. This is for good reason. If something goes unexpectedly wrong before, during or immediately after an operation, as a result of surgical or anaesthetic complications or even a poorly patient, we may have only seconds to assess and rectify a situation before there are serious consequences. For example, the endotracheal tube (ETT). This is the hollow silicone tube that passes from your lips, past your tongue, through your vocal cords and into the trachea (windpipe). It allows the anaesthetist to provide oxygen and ventilate the lungs of an unconscious patient. I talk about it a lot. In an adult, if an ETT dislodges during surgery, or we have difficulty placing it in position in the first place, you may have only one or two minutes to replace it before the patient suffers a cardiac arrest. If a baby's ETT falls out, you may only have

---

12 That is not a joke!

30 seconds. We run over these imaginary scenarios time and time again. We train in simulated operating room environments where we practise running through clinical management algorithms to treat various potentially serious events. This is a sort of repetitive, rote-learning environment to prime us for recognition and almost automatic response to various scenarios.

Let me use an example: managing anaphylaxis. Anaphylaxis is a hypersensitivity reaction to a drug or food. We administer many intravenous drugs in the operating theatre, all of which carry a risk of anaphylaxis – all drugs do. An awake person may be able to tell you they are feeling itchy, feeling faint or, dangerously, having difficulty breathing as an indicator of anaphylaxis. But when you are anaesthetised, you lose any ability to communicate. You won't be aware or recall having had anaphylaxis, but the astute anaesthetist must be tuned in to other signs that may suggest it: tachycardia (a high heart-rate), hypotension (low blood-pressure), bronchospasm (tightening of the airways) or a distinctive rash. The problem is, these signs are not unique to anaphylaxis. You may be tachycardic because we haven't given enough pain relief yet, or you may have low blood-pressure, as there is slightly too much anaesthetic drug in your system at that point. This is where the simulated environment comes into its own. It is a fully functional theatre environment using sophisticated manikins that can have their vital signs manipulated by the devious tutors operating the system behind one-way glass. You, the trainee, walk in, knowing full well something horrible is about to happen to the forgiving manikin, all while being observed by your peers. It teaches you to make rapid assessments, think of what might be happening and make quick clinical decisions once you have diagnosed the problem. In this example, once anaphylaxis is recognised, the algorithms act as a reminder of the appropriate immediate treatment: securing the airway before it closes over, adrenalin, steroids, intravenous fluid and cessation of the offending drug if it is still being given. We are trained to expect the unexpected. I don't want to terrify anyone, as these scenarios are rare (after ten years working in anaes-thesia, I am yet to manage an intraoperative anaphylaxis), but anaes-thetists do have to handle them.

After a few months as an anaesthetic SHO, I could see why we used to see them as 'shit-cool bastards'. However awful a clinical scenario seemed to me as a junior intern on the wards, the anaes-thetist had always seen and dealt with worse in the operating thea-tre or ICU. There is an old saying in anaesthesia circles that the job is 95 per cent boredom and 5 per cent blind panic. 'Blind panic' might be an overstatement – 5 per cent squeaky-bum time might be more apt. This is why we occasionally get the reputation for being pedantic or over-cautious; we want to sit back and embrace bore-dom in the operating room.

There is a steep learning curve in anaesthesia training. On day one, you are completely useless. You are unable to bag-mask venti-late a patient (the most crucial and basic skill in anaesthesia used to squeeze air into the lungs of an unconscious person). You cannot put in a large cannula. You certainly cannot intubate anyone (the process of inserting an ETT). Don't even think about attempting something advanced like an epidural. You spend the first week struggling, under constant supervision, wondering if you'll ever get the hang of it. Then all of a sudden, you begin to master these basic skills. After three or four months, you are capable of delivering a simple, safe anaesthetic to a very low-risk patient. You gain confi-dence quickly to the point where you think this is all plain sailing, and then – bang. One of those unexpected events happens, except you weren't expecting it, because you're not experienced. A pull of the emergency bell or a call for help and a senior registrar or a consultant comes and bails you out.[13] It is frightening, but the

---

13 Most theatre departments are equipped with emergency buzzers in each operating room that sound out to summon help when a critical situation arises.

wake-up call gives you a better appreciation for the skills of the senior anaesthetists and just how crucial it is to be vigilant at all times.

My 'bang' moment came four months into training when an adult patient slid halfway off the operating table during the operation. I dived across the floor faster than Peter Schmeichel to prevent his head bouncing off the floor. The error, it turned out, was that the safety straps had not been secured properly. This isn't necessarily the specific duty of the anaesthetist, but ultimately we are responsible for all aspects of patient safety in theatre. I always check the safety straps myself since that day. I'd like to retire without having to make a cranium-saving dive ever again.

Although all anaesthesia is based on the same themes and principles, there are nuances to providing anaesthesia for one type of surgery over another. Anaesthesia for neurosurgery is similar to, but not exactly the same as, anaesthesia for orthopaedic surgery, for example. Anaesthesia for abdominal surgery is similar to, but not exactly the same as, anaesthesia for ear, nose and throat (ENT) and so on. The factors we consider before determining what sort of anaesthetic to provide broadly come into two categories: patient factors and surgical factors, and how they interact. For example, we need to have very tight blood pressure control in neurosurgery in order to adequately perfuse the brain but also minimise the risk of catastrophic bleeding in the brain. This is less of an issue in, say, general surgery. If a patient has several severe comorbid conditions making a general anaesthetic risky then we can consider if the operation can be performed under regional anaesthesia (for example, a spinal anaesthetic or nerve block – more on these later). Orthopaedic surgery is very suited to this, whereas it is almost impossible in ENT surgery.

Obstetric anaesthesia, though, is consistently different. In my second year of training I worked in obstetric anaesthesia where you learn to work fast. You have to. A ward full of labouring women is extremely dynamic, with clinical scenarios changing rapidly (the screams add to the drama, of course). Epidural in Room 4. Caesarean section in Theatre 2. Epidural in Room 5. Epidural in Room 8. The epidural in Room 4 isn't working well. Caesarean section in Theatre 2. Epidural in Room 2. Post-partum haemorrhage in Room 1. Epidural top-up in Room 8. Retained placenta in Theatre 1. This goes on and on, night after night. I worked every third night for six months in my obstetric rotation. I can't remember if I slept. I think I did. We competed to see who could get out of bed, run down to the labour ward, place an epidural and get back to bed in the fastest time. We needed all the sleep we could get. Twelve minutes was my record. You become adept at managing emergencies, but the hours were diabolical. I sometimes worked 100 hours in a week and had no time to spend any of the overtime money. In a fugue-like, sleep-deprived state, I bought a car with cash at the end of the six-month posting. It was a flashy white coupé. A senior registrar told me I looked like a drug dealer. I guess I am, in a way.

If obstetric anaesthesia tires you out, intensive care medicine grinds you down and tests your resolve. Anaesthetists in training tend to spend the bulk of their middle years (three to four of six) working in the ICU. I had initially pursued anaesthesia training as a means to becoming an intensivist (an intensive care physician). I loved being the ICU registrar when the ED would call for help in the resuscitation room when a critically ill person arrived in an ambulance with its raging blue lights on. It was so fast paced and exciting. They needed my skills. Rapidly assess. Resuscitate. Intubate. Arrange ICU bed. Place central line and arterial line. Talk to family. Transfer to CT scan. Transfer to ICU. Choose antibiotics. Start dialysis. Support the heart. It was literally all the things I had previously decided my ideal job would be. The shit-cool bastard, cool as a cucumber. But night after night of putting out fires in the ED, on wards and in the ICU leaves one a little numb. It never stops. There are so many critically unwell patients all over our hospitals and nowhere near enough ICU beds for them all. Some poor patients sit in our ICUs and don't make any progress for months on end, if any at all. It started to wear down my patience and, worse, my empathy. This is a red flag for a doctor, a warning sign for burnout. I thought I should reconsider intensive care as my long-term career choice.

By the time you become a senior anaesthesia registrar, you have seen a lot and been in enough squirmy situations to be confident that you can safely manage most scenarios. There are still things beyond your abilities, but you have access to anaesthesia and intensive care consultants who can help you make the big decisions. But the deeper you move into your training, the more responsibility you accept. You are now the 'senior registrar' on call, which means that you are the most senior anaesthetist in the hospital at night and often the most senior doctor in the entire hospital at night. Depending on where you work, you could be supervising up to three more junior anaesthetists on a night shift. I say 'night shift', but this can be anything from 12 to 30 hours depending on which hospital one works in.[14] There might be an SHO in the operating theatre, an SHO or registrar in the maternity unit and another registrar in the ICU. You are expected to risk assess everything that is going on and place yourself in a position to help the junior that needs it most at any given moment. It's a lot of responsibility, especially when two critical situations are going on simultaneously; say, an emergency Caesarean section in a high-risk patient, a critically unwell child in the ED, a severe head trauma that needs emergency neurosurgery – risk assess, risk assess, risk assess. You can call the consultant at home for advice of course, but some things need to be

---

14 Although we are supposed to be entirely compliant with the EU Working Time Directive (EWTD), it is a fact that many doctors still work ludicrously long shifts due to rota gaps and some resistance to change from those who did work ridiculous hours 'back in the day'. It is improving, slowly.

dealt with immediately. Confidence in your abilities comes with experience, and by the end of a year as a senior registrar you start to feel like a consultant.

All trainee anaesthetists must spend time in a specialised children's hospital to gain experience caring for and anaesthetising babies and other children with particular paediatric problems. Generally, only more experienced trainees rotate through the children's hospitals because it is not the place to be learning your basic anaesthesia skills. The stakes are higher. You are not only treating a patient who may not be able to verbalise their problems but also the parents who may not be able to grasp what is wrong with their child either. From a technical perspective, most tasks that are easy in an adult are significantly trickier in a baby or child. It can be hard to cannulate a vein that is only 2 mm in diameter.

I had been leaning towards a future in adult intensive care medicine, but that idea was shelved when I had my first rotation in a children's hospital. The environment is totally different. Everyone goes by first names, all the time. This breaks down hierarchical barriers. Everyone is available, all the time. Consultants in a paediatric environment are always happy to be called in the middle of the night and will be available in person in a flash if their presence is required at 3 a.m. This ensures the best care always occurs. Everyone does what is best for the child, all the time. The positivity was so refreshing. Almost immediately, I knew the career that would give me both the greatest challenges and the most satisfaction was that of a paediatric anaesthetist.

Paediatric Anaesthetist

I returned to the same paediatric hospital I had worked in as a junior registrar for my sixth and final year of anaesthesia training. By this point I was 100 per cent certain that I wanted a career working exclusively in paediatric anaesthesia. Children are phenomenal creatures. They are so resilient, so strong. When they become critically unwell, they have an unbelievable ability to bounce back and recover. At the time of writing, I have no children of my own, but I can only imagine the anxiety a parent must feel as they hand over their child to the care of a complete stranger. We as paediatric doctors are in a uniquely privileged position to be trusted in such a way.

The final year of anaesthesia training is strange. You are so close to the end, you feel like your skills are almost at consultant level, yet the goal of securing a consultant post still seems unattainable. It makes sense to feel that way – the competition is fierce. As you and your peers enter the final year of training, you can sense the tension knowing 40 other anaesthetists each year will be scrambling out of the assault course, covered in mud, clutching their Certificate of Completion of Specialist Training (CCST) making you eligible to apply for consultant jobs. But, with few attractive consultant jobs to apply for, there can be a lot of jostling for position. The uncertainty is jarring: *I've been training for 16 years and I could be on the dole in four months' time.*

Most trainees try to spend their final year of training in a hospital where they would like to work as a consultant in the long run. It's like a year-long job interview. The pressure is on not only to complete your education but at the same time to try to prove your particular worth to the department. You want to demonstrate that you will be tolerable to work with for the next 30 years. Any small slip-up can make it seem like you've blown your chances.

In my final year, an email circulated from the registrar who was in charge of our daily roster informing us that we may need to make changes to the working day as the paediatric ICU (PICU) consultants were concerned that our ward rounds were finishing too late. Safe in the knowledge that I was in a private discussion with my peers, I vented that the real reason we were usually late finishing was because 'the PICU consultants need to get the finger out and start the rounds on time'. Reply all, send. *Beep beep. Beep beep. Beep beep.* Three WhatsApp messages in a row? Strange. Three different trainees – 'Colin, you know the consultants are in that email thread?' *Oh shit. Why? WHY?! They never are! Shit, shit, shit. Well that's it, Colin, you're never getting a job in this hospital.* I decided that the best course of action was to be honest. I would stick to my guns as, although this hadn't been the best way to bring it up, I genuinely felt this was the reason we weren't going home until 8 p.m. some nights. I sent a follow-up email apologising for my tone, but reinforcing my point and insisting I was speaking on behalf of my peers. *Beep beep* – a text from a PICU consultant. 'Colin, I completely agree with you.' Oh, sweet relief.

Irish consultants are among the best trained in the world. We have post-graduate training programmes that are not only longer than other jurisdictions, but broader. This means most Irish trainees, when they get to the end of training, have significantly more experience than many other countries. Our longer working hours add many extra hours to this experience also, for better or worse. So, how do you stand out when there's a new consultant job advertised? Even more training, that's how. *Supra*-specialised training. Imagine Superman going back to do a PhD in chemical engineering to *really* get an understanding of Kryptonite. Or Roger Federer learning how to carve his own tennis rackets. Further subspecialty training is called a fellowship: a fully trained specialist, consultant-level doctor goes (usually) abroad for an additional year or two of supra-specialised training to become even more expert in an even narrower field. This might be, for example, in robotic cancer surgery for a urologist,[15] in interventional cardiology for a cardiologist, or in obstetric anaesthesia for an anaesthetist. This is technically not a requisite to gain a consultant post, but if you are to land one in Ireland you better have at least one fellowship (if not two, or even

---

15 This does not mean cancer in robots.

three in some specialties) and perhaps even a PhD to go along with it.[16] In fact, there are many superb, well-trained Irish doctors abroad who were snapped up by the hospitals in North America, Australia and the UK where they went for this further training and, sadly for Irish patients, elected to stay abroad.[17]

Knowing this, I decided to combine two of my favourite subjects – cardiology and paediatric anaesthesia. Paediatric cardiac anaesthetist. *This title is becoming a mouthful.* I applied to the world-famous Great Ormond Street Hospital (GOSH) in London. With only one cardiac anaesthesia fellowship available each year, I didn't fancy my chances. I gazed up at the weary red-brick façade of the hospital one cold November day, nervously tapping my cup of undrunk coffee as I waited, the history and significance of the hospital oozing from the walls. Expecting to be invited into a grand boardroom to be interviewed by 15 Charles Darwin lookalikes, I was surprised to be crammed into a tiny room with a much less intimidating group of three – and disappointingly, not a single bearded Victorian gent among them.

I defied my own expectations and received a call telling me I had been successful shortly after the interview. The post was for 18 months in London working in all things heart related. My wife got great news too. She made a bold move and asked to be temporarily

---

16 Instead of a PhD, I chose to do a master's degree which I completed … with my own money (€17k) … in my spare time … in between anaesthesia exams … during my anaesthesia training … sometimes working 80+ hours per week.

17 There are several reasons for this, but this not being a politically motivated book I will only mention them briefly. A chronic shortage of consultants exists in Ireland but in order to reach the tipping point and attract people back to Ireland, a number of things must occur. Guaranteed additional resources to effectively run services, more inpatient hospital beds, government investment in areas of need and pay parity. Consultants appointed after 2012 earn up to 50 per cent *less* than those hired before 2012. For doing the exact same job. You read that correctly.

released from her surgical training programme in Ireland. They granted her one year out of her training programme, and she landed a fantastic job in central London. We were very fortunate.

Paediatric Cardiac Anaesthetist

Working at GOSH is the paediatric medicine equivalent of playing in the Champions League. It is one of the most famous hospitals in the world. Experts from all over the world come to work and carry out research there. It is steeped in history. Charles Dickens, a former local resident, organised annual fundraising 'Anniversary Festivals' from 1852 onwards and was also known to perform readings of *A Christmas Carol* in order to raise funds to keep the hospital running. J. M. Barrie gifted the copyright to *Peter Pan* to the hospital in 1929 and they still benefit from this today. Understandably, GOSH staff are immensely proud of the heritage of this grand old institution.

The cardiac department is the biggest paediatric cardiac department in the UK and one of the biggest in Europe, taking many international referrals. Arriving as a foreign graduate and having trained as an anaesthetist abroad, it suddenly struck me that maybe they did things completely differently here. *What if I do something that they think is stupid? Maybe they have some wonder drug I've never heard of. What if their anaesthetic technique includes reading excerpts from* Peter Pan? I was slightly standoffish at first in order to observe their practice before coming to the conclusion that it was fundamentally the same as in Ireland. Safe in the knowledge that the practice of anaesthesia was almost universal, and that I would not make an arse of myself, I could focus on getting the necessary experience. They were very welcoming. It was noted that I said 'grand' a lot and called all the children 'pet'. It was also noted that my wife was a trainee urologist – 'How's the cock doctor, Colin?' I would be asked. Strange, I thought, she's a 'dick doctor' in Ireland. These were the first of many linguistic curiosities I'd note were different from my Hiberno-English.

In London, we performed many of the same operations as in Ireland but with a few additional procedures, like heart transplants. I won't forget the first heart transplant I witnessed in a child. I gazed over the surgical drapes and fixated on this cavernous hole in the centre of the child's chest, where their heart used to lie. There was a person in front of me with no heart in their chest.[18] The old, damaged heart could not go back in. They would be dead if the new one didn't function. Think how strange that sounds. I watched as the surgeon placed the final sutures before re-perfusing the new heart (reintroducing blood flow). A few minutes passed. Nothing. I was concerned, but no one else seemed to be. Then suddenly, a flicker of movement, slow at first, like a muscle twitch. A new squiggle on the ECG tracing. Nothing you would call 'normal', but some electrical activity. Then more movement, more vigorous now. Ten minutes later and the heart, that just four hours ago was inside another, now sadly deceased, human being, in another part of the country, was now pumping in a new home. It defies logic. Throughout that year in London, seeing this phenomenon never lost its magic. Every time I saw a patient given a new lease of life with the most generous of donations from another person, I would stop for a moment to soak it in. How privileged I was to be a part of it.

My astute mother-in-law ensured that I did not miss the advertisement for a consultant paediatric anaesthetist post in Dublin. The stakes were high. By this stage, my wife had already moved back to Ireland to continue her surgical training in Galway. With four more years of her training to go, I had to land the job to even live in the same country as my wife. If I failed, then I would be in limbo in a situation where I was living in the UK, possibly working

---

18 They are kept alive using cardiopulmonary bypass; more on that later.

as a consultant in the NHS, impatiently wondering when, if ever, the next consultant post would be available for me in Ireland. We had always envisioned our lives in Ireland in the long run. If I did not land the job, the hypothetical scenario where my wife (and any future children) would move permanently to the UK would become slightly more realistic. This would not only massively disrupt her training, but would also be hard on our close family. The catch was that after my time in London, I was now probably so specialised in paediatric cardiac anaesthesia that I could only reasonably expect to get a consultant post in this single specialised hospital in Ireland. All the eggs in one disinfected, MRSA-free, hospital basket.

There were two consultant anaesthetist jobs available but of course many more applicants. The pressure was on. At this point, impostor syndrome sets in. It's hard to picture yourself as a consultant when you have been taught by so many excellent consultants over the years. You start to second-guess your credentials. *Am I really qualified to do this? Is my CV good enough? Have I published enough research? Am I clinically ready to be entirely independent? Will my references be supportive?*

My interview was one of those exams in which none of the subjects you studied get asked, touching on about 3 per cent of what I had prepared. Clearly, terrified that I would be tongue-tied in the interview, I had over-prepared. *But what if they ask about this?* The fear of having nothing to say left me, an expert in useless trivia about the history of the health service, familiar with the names of the first quintuplets born in Ireland and how much the minister for health spends on socks each year.

Post-interview, as my father drove me back to Dublin airport to return to London, my phone rang. The interview panel seemingly liked what they had heard, as the news was positive. My dad cheered like he would when Manchester United scored yet another injury-time winner. I called my wife; she was in tears on the other side of the country. There was no time to celebrate as I boarded a flight back to London to get to GOSH in time for my night shift. I was still a registrar in name, but at least my future was now secure. Relief.

So that's how you become an anaesthetist.

PART 2

Observations of an Anaesthetist

A switch does not flick once you become a consultant. You have only one more day's experience than the day before. And the day before you were a registrar or a fellow. All that has changed is the title on your ID badge. Consultants do not know everything. A solicitor cannot recite the entire constitution. A concert pianist cannot play every concerto perfectly. Medicine evolves and practice changes. We have a duty to continue our education, and it doesn't end when you reach the end of your formal training. Consultants are obliged to attend regular courses and conferences to keep up to date. We don't have all the answers and we too are constantly learning and our practice evolving.

The first year in a consultant post is a daunting prospect. Your head is still filled with the uncertainties. You still second-guess your credentials. All eyes are on you. Because I felt it would be a monumental year in my career, I chose to document it.

I have never kept a diary before. This was initially an exercise for myself to remember and reflect on what I assumed would be some of my most memorable days in clinical medicine. However, it quickly became clear to me that my mood and lasting memories on any given day were intensely influenced by my interactions with other staff or patients, or observing other people interacting. You cannot avoid this when working in an operating theatre, the beating heart of the hospital, full of animated characters.

On the flipside to this, I could see that I could greatly influence the mood of children and parents coming to theatre. They hang on every word, so they must be chosen carefully. You would be surprised at the seemingly trivial things that patients get apprehensive about. The method in which I crafted and delivered my explanation of a child's journey into the operating room and undergoing anaesthesia could significantly alter their expectations. It is an important interaction. It is rewarding, then, to feel that palpable anxiety dissipate when I get an explanation just right. I pondered the question: what do people really know about anaesthesia?

So, after a couple of weeks of writing a personal diary, it became an intentional explanation of what anaesthesia is, what goes on in the operating theatre and what the evolving life of a new consultant anaesthetist in a children's hospital is all about.

1 – Pulling Teeth

For me, it feels as if I never left. The return of my familiar face, however, gives rise to looks of horror as people question what they have been doing with their lives over the 21 months since they saw me last.

'Has it been that long?'

'I'm afraid so.'

'Why did you come back?'

Why would a consultant return to a chaotic health system that is chronically understaffed, under-resourced and bursting at the seams? A job in which, in some cases, I will earn almost 50 per cent less than a senior colleague for doing the same day-to-day work? Where staff are so undervalued that they resort to strike action? The answer is simple. I am overwhelmingly thankful for my medical education and the anaesthesia training I received, from the Irish taxpayer, that I feel duty bound and obliged to use what I know for the benefit of the Irish population, as best I can. London was just finishing school, but Ireland is home. Naturally, my answer to the above question ran more along the lines of, 'You know yourself, the wife is working in Galway, so I had to come back.'

The first day back in the job and I have what has been occasionally dubbed the 'mental dental' list. This is due to the volume and complexity of cases booked in for dental operations.[1] The dental surgeon may be performing simple extractions or complex restorations. Most of the children on our dental lists have complex medical problems, some degree of learning disability or severe behavioural issues. Parents struggle to maintain oral hygiene in this group of kids. The process of inducing anaesthesia is often the most taxing part of the child's journey through the dental theatre. Even getting them into the anaesthetic room is like pulling teeth. Our dental surgeon, though, is expert in managing challenging children.

The major challenge of the day is anaesthetising a young teenager with severe autism who weighed nearly 20 kg more than me. Unfortunately, he has been known to get aggressive at times, particularly when he is in unfamiliar surroundings. He could easily knock me out with a rogue elbow. To make this process as seamless as possible, we agree with his mother to give him a sedating premedication in the day ward before coming to theatre. Premedication is

---

1 To avoid any confusion or offence, I must point out that 'mental' is analogous to 'chaotic' when referencing this theatre list. It is busy for the anaesthetist and extremely challenging. It is not 'mental' in the sense of an outdated Victorian descriptor of those with mental illness.

normal practice for particularly anxious children pre-operatively. To keep him calm, we expel all but essential personnel from the theatre itself and turn the lights down to keep it as peaceful as possible. However, we must make contingency plans if he gets upset, as we also have to keep the safety of the staff high on our agenda. We elect to have a dummy run in theatre so everyone knows what role they will play. Our petite dental surgeon hops on the trolley and assumes the role of the patient. She gives it her best shot but is no match for two burly porters who gently and safely restrain her as if they were dragging her away from the cake in the tea room. *That's enough now.*

Our patient arrives and we learn he refused to take his prescribed sedatives, preferring to chuck them on the floor in delight. His mother looks concerned. We hadn't planned for this. We were trying to avoid needles as he has previously not been too happy with the prospect of an IV cannula, but in someone his size, with no sedative on board, it's probably the easiest thing to do. With an IV in place, we can very rapidly induce anaesthesia intravenously compared to the relatively slow onset of anaesthesia using gas in a large patient. The porters step forward as if to ready themselves for the stare-off before a world championship boxing match. But I get the feeling the patient is actually not too concerned today. He makes no eye contact with anyone, typical of severe autism, but allows me to take his hand and plunge the needle in to the back of it. With that in place, inducing anaesthesia is easy. No contingency plans required today.

2 – Stress, Fear, Anxiety

Stress. Fear. Anxiety. Today, on just my second day in the job, I felt what it is truly like to be a consultant. As a trainee you have a comfort blanket around you, knowing that there is a superior to advise you, to make the tough decisions and to guide you with their experience[2] – which can lull you into a false sense of security. Fast forward a mere few months: you're the consultant, making the tough decisions. Crucially, there's a difference between thinking like a consultant and actually acting like one, and this is where your lack of experience in the role can show.

A neonate is any baby less than a month old. Healthy babies, born at term, do occasionally need surgery. Neonatal anaesthesia is tough; it's the deep end of the swimming pool.[3] However, those born prematurely – especially at less than 30 weeks' gestation – are practically a different species. Never mind the swimming pool, this is jumping into the Mariana Trench. Unfortunately, due to their prematurity, this group often have multiple medical problems that warrant surgical interventions. They are also tough to anaesthetise; their lung and heart functions have so little in reserve that things can go downhill very quickly if you are not hyper-vigilant. In some ways, although congenital heart disease and paediatric heart surgery can scare anaesthetists, it is ultimately formulaic. Every baby gets the same package of care – the same type of anaesthetic and a cardiopulmonary bypass machine ready and waiting for every case. That is my comfort zone, having spent the last 18 months working in that field. However, a sick preemie requiring

---

2 Now writing as a consultant, I use the term 'trainee' as a general catch-all descriptor for any doctor who is not a consultant. 'Junior doctor' or 'non-consultant hospital doctor' (NCHD) are the same thing and come under my 'trainee' umbrella. Most of the anaesthesia 'trainees' in a paediatric hospital are actually quite senior registrars, so don't make the assumption that they are complete novices.

3 You will notice I talk about gestation in weeks as opposed to months, as this is standard vernacular in the hospital. 'Full term' is 40 weeks, or 9 months. A 'term' baby is any born over 37 weeks' gestation. Everything before that is technically premature; however, there is a vast difference in a premature baby born at 36 weeks and one born at 24 weeks. We often use the term 'ex-prem' to describe a slightly older child who was born prematurely or a 'preemie' to describe a premature neonate.

major abdominal surgery is not. *I know the principles, I have the skills.*

Something you are aware of, but not particularly bothered by as a trainee, is the impression the surgeon has of you and your practice. As the anaesthetist, your speed in inducing anaesthesia, inserting whatever monitoring lines you need and performing a regional block, before whisking the patient into the operating room from the adjoining anaesthetic room, is a rate-limiting factor for the surgeon.[4] Many surgeons would operate all day (and possibly all night) if they were allowed, and so they might think that a fast anaesthetist is a good anaesthetist – an attitude typical of an adult hospital. Children's hospitals are different. Everyone appreciates the difficulty of working on a neonate. Nevertheless, as the new consultant, you want to impress your surgical colleagues. You want them to rate you: this guy was good, he kept the list moving, there were no delays. Nobody trains us for this.

Today's baby weighs less than 2kg, and was born extremely prematurely.[5] She was born with a major abdominal abnormality,

---

4 Regional anaesthesia is a method of anaesthesia where an injection of local anaesthetic solution is performed with the aim of anaesthetising specific nerves that supply the area being operated on. It is usually performed with the help of an ultrasound machine. The local anaesthesia temporarily blocks nerve transmission so the patient will feel little or no pain. Surgery in adults can be performed entirely under regional anaesthesia or a 'nerve block' as it is sometimes called. An epidural is an example of a commonly performed regional anaesthesia technique. It is possible in children but it is more common for us to combine regional anaesthesia with a general anaesthetic as asking a four-year-old to sit still while surgery is performed is as successful as leaving the dog to mind the Christmas turkey.

5 If a baby is born at 28 weeks and is now 4 weeks old we would describe them as 32 weeks corrected gestational age (CGA). It is useful to use CGA as it gives us an idea of what stage of development the baby is at. A baby born at 24 weeks could be 3 months old but still only 36 weeks CGA and thus not as developed as a full-term baby. You're now ready to sit your paediatric exams – good luck.

a major cardiac abnormality and lung disease associated with prematurity. She has yet to leave the walls of the hospital. She has not yet managed to breathe without some help from a ventilator. Some start. To add to this, she has an abnormal airway. One of the basic tenets of anaesthesia is successfully intubating a patient's trachea. It is almost always straightforward but, on occasion, it can be very difficult, or impossible. We can usually predict who is going to have a 'difficult airway' and plan accordingly. In babies, a difficult airway is usually associated with a number of specific syndromes. This means the process of inducing anaesthesia will be extremely hazardous. This is before we even get to surgery, which can't take place until we have overcome this hurdle. She is here for major abdominal surgery. 'Please discuss your management plan for this case.' If this were a case in the anaesthesia examinations, students would complain that it was unrealistic.

It would have been nice to have a week of easy anaesthesia to kick off my consultant career but, alas, here we are. I seek out a senior colleague for advice, but we're short on the ground and everyone is tied up. Nobody wants to make a balls of something in their first week, but I'm on my own. I make a mental plan. Be quick, keep everyone happy. The baby has a difficult course in the operating theatre, but she gets through the operation and we return her to the paediatric intensive care unit (PICU). I am relieved, but not happy. My internal monologue is in overdrive. *You should've done this. You shouldn't have done that. Or should you? You will next time. Or will you?*

A gap in the operating list in the afternoon allows me to follow up on her in PICU. To my horror, I see a lot of activity around her bed and the PICU consultants working hard to stabilise her. She has not been doing well since I left her. I want the ground to swallow me up. Stress. Fear. Anxiety. *What did you miss? What did you do?* I return an hour later to check again, and she's in better condition but by no means perfect. I can feel the eyes on me, I can hear the whispers. The personal feeling that I could have done a better job is confounded by the feeling of being judged by my consultant peers. When you hand over a critically unwell patient to another doctor, you cannot help but think that their current clinical status, in all its sickly ugliness, is entirely your fault. It's easy to forget that they were poorly to begin with and have had, in the interim, a major surgical assault on their tiny little body. In all probability, the baby would have been unstable regardless of what I did, as she was so unwell, but it's impossible not to worry that more senior consultants might think me naïve or, worse, incapable for my choices, all because of this one case, on my second day.

Or, stepping back, is this the dreaded impostor syndrome? Feeling incompetent and useless, despite being well trained and highly skilled. There was no bad outcome for the baby and I hadn't made any mistakes, but I couldn't shake the sense that I could have done more to deliver a 'less sick' patient to the ICU. The desire to be accepted as one of the team in theatre affected my better judgement. I was blinkered to the bigger picture. I tell myself it won't happen again. Or maybe no one was judging me at all.

I suffer a minor existential crisis that evening driving to Galway to see my wife. *Do you know the principles? Do you have the skills? Are you good enough to do this job?* My wife, in her surgical capacity, gives me an appreciation for how a surgeon feels every time they go home in the evening. Relentless ruminations: 'Have I damaged the bowel?' 'Will the patient be ok?' 'Am I able to do this operation?' 'What if they're bleeding?' I don't know how she sleeps at night. I decide I am good enough and accept that it was a challenging case that many would have struggled with. But I have learned a valuable lesson – there is no substitute for experience and this day will be forever logged in the memory bank.

5 – Narcos

There are many drugs in a hospital pharmacy. Hundreds, if not thousands, available at any one time. They range from various over-the-counter medications like paracetamol, which cost mere pennies, all the way up the scale to new-fangled, hi-tech, cutting-edge drugs that are revolutionising treatment for some chronic diseases and cancers. These can cost tens of thousands. Per dose. But just because some medications are cheap doesn't mean they're ineffective. When a drug goes 'off-patent', after a number of years, any pharmaceutical company can produce that drug, and thus the price plummets. These are known as generic drugs. The years 'on patent' are when the manufacturers aim to recoup all the money they piled into research and development, plus a tidy profit. If paracetamol was invented now, it would be a gold mine.

Generic drugs are essentially all we use in anaesthesia and, despite the fact they are old, they are still phenomenal drugs. I guarantee you, every drug ever used as an anaesthetic agent would still knock you out today. Anaesthetics of the past, like chloroform or ether, would still render the modern man unconscious. Even enough alcohol would do the trick, but we have moved on. As medicine progresses, we become more discerning in what we consider to be a useful drug. We want an anaesthetic drug to knock you out, but with minimal hangover; to knock you out, but with no effect on other organs; to knock you out, but with no side effects. Therefore, the palate of drugs that we use on a daily basis is really quite small. We have access to many drugs, but the core of our anaesthetic recipe consists of maybe fewer than five medications.

The drugs that we rely on are immensely powerful, but immensely dangerous. If an untrained person were to administer our drugs, it would almost certainly lead to extreme morbidity (an aspiration pneumonia at best or a cardiac arrest at worst) or even death. The lethal injection in the United States consists of thiopentone, potassium chloride and pancuronium – all drugs that you will find in the anaesthetist's drawer, which aren't lethal when used in the trained hands of an anaesthetist who is ready to take over the breathing of an unconscious patient.

At the very core of anaesthesia is pain relief, and although we have made great progress with regional anaesthesia, our most potent IV pain relievers are still from the opiate family. The opiates are derived from the opium plant and are probably the oldest anaesthetic drugs in the world.[6] Opium derivatives have been used, and abused, for centuries, morphine being the most common. These drugs bind to opiate receptors in the body and give the recipient feelings of immense pain relief, but also sedation and euphoria. Too much, though, and you will stop breathing. It is this side effect that kills so many illicit opiate users from overdoses of heroin and fentanyl (a synthetic, super-potent opioid), amongst others.

The opioid crisis in the United States has taken a turn for the worse in recent decades as masses of super-potent fentanyl has flooded the illicit market. It is extremely easy to overdose, yet we administer this drug multiple times per day. Legitimately. We administer these drugs so frequently that I sometimes forget that the patient is probably experiencing something they will never experience again, unless they embark on a career of illicit drug abuse. Fentanyl is regularly administered as part of an intravenous induction in advance of propofol.[7] For those few moments between receiving fentanyl and the propofol rendering the patient uncon-

---

6 Although technically not an anaesthetic drug, it is an analgesic drug. Analgesic means pain reliever. An opioid is a synthetic drug that binds to opiate receptors whereas opiates are drugs naturally derived from the opium plant. They have the same effects, more or less.

7 Fentanyl is colourless, while propofol looks like milk. This distinction led a surgeon to summarise anaesthesia practice to me: 'What is there to anaesthesia? Just give clear stuff, then white stuff.'

scious, they may be experiencing utterly glorious, opioid-induced euphoria.

The little girl I anaesthetised today arrived in theatre with her mother and an IV cannula already in place. I flushed the cannula with some saline to make sure it was working. Propofol can sting, so pushing it through a dodgy cannula is not advised. Everything seemed to be in order, so I fired through a standard dose of fentanyl for her weight into the cannula. Reaching for the propofol, I dropped the syringe on the ground and had to toss it in the bin. I sauntered over to our drug trolley to draw up more, returning to the patient's side about 30 seconds later. At this point, she turned to her mother, beaming from ear to ear.

'Is this what drugs feel like?! Am I high? Woooowwwwww!'

The fentanyl had hit her. Her mother turned to look at me with an expression that suggested I had just condemned her daughter to a lifetime of hard-core intravenous drug abuse, prostitution and burglary. I rapidly pushed in the propofol and she went to sleep. The concerned mother enquired, 'Will she be ok after … that?' I assumed she meant, 'Do I need to seek help for opioid dependency?' I smiled and reassured her this was a totally normal response to the drugs.

This is not the first time I've had a reaction such as this as an anaesthetist. As I slowly emptied a syringe of propofol into a respectable-looking professional, he smiled and proclaimed, 'This is better than *any* gear I've ever done!' Worrying. We also use ketamine in anaesthesia both to induce anaesthesia and, at much lower doses, for chronic pain. Ketamine is now a leading drug of abuse. I recall receiving a call from a consultant when I was a trainee to go to a ward to see one of his chronic pain patients. The instructions were to give her a small dose of IV ketamine to see if it had any effect. This pleasant forty-something lady seemed to be suffering, barely acknowledging me as I attempted introductions. Knowing it was not standard practice to be dosing people with IV ketamine on the wards, I elected to administer a minuscule dose first, about 25 per cent of what the consultant instructed me to, just in case. No effect. I waited ten minutes and repeated the tiny dose. Nothing. I walked out to the nurses' station to write a note in her chart. Seconds later, a student nurse called out from the door. 'Excuse me, there's a woman in here saying she's panicking from ketamine or something?' I peered in and my patient was sitting up, eyes wide open. She saw me and pulled me by the scruff of the neck into a deep embrace.

'That was ketamine?' she asked.

'Yes, it was. Are you ok?'

'I used to take loads of ketamine and it never did this! Am I dying?'

'No, you're not dying!'

'THANK YOU, THANK YOU, THANK YOU!'

After several more sweaty embraces I injected her with some midazolam to calm her down and returned to complete my note in the chart:

Patient extremely sensitive to ketamine administration. No pain reported after dosing; however, she is demonstrating acute ketamine intoxication. Not suitable as long-term treatment for her chronic pain.

8 – The Factory Floor

Not all anaesthesia is thought provoking, cognitively challenging and a test of your technical skills. Sometimes we are there to provide a service only and work full steam ahead to help churn through high-volume lists. Today is one of those days. We are working with the dermatologists who perform laser procedures to remove various skin lesions such as 'port wine stains' or *nevus flammeus*. The majority of these kids are generally healthy, with the exception of the skin abnormality. The procedure can take up to 20 minutes, and it stings.

Eleven patients on the list, four hours to do it all. We operate a conveyor-belt-like system: I anaesthetise a child in the operating theatre, and the next one arrives in the anaesthetic room. My registrar anaesthetises the child in the adjoining anaesthetic room, and as soon as the procedure finishes inside, we are ready to roll with the next one. As we wheel patient two into theatre, patient three arrives in the anaesthetic room, and so the pattern goes on. Our trainees have been with us for a month now, and are starting to get comfortable anaesthetising children. So we install a tag-team tactic: I do one case, the registrar does the next. It keeps us moving and gives the trainee some independence while I am close by.

In contrast to adult practice, children generally are anaesthetised by inhaling anaesthetic gas via a mask held over their nose and mouth. There are no hard-and-fast rules as to when to switch over to an IV technique, but the pain and distress of getting a needle poked into the skin is probably greater than that of using the mask, and we might have to poke them repeatedly; it's hard to hit a 2-millimetre vein when the target is upset and squirming.[8]

Anaesthetists and nurses new to paediatric practice notice the anaesthetic gas a lot. The stuff smells pretty pungent. While we try our best to have the child breathing most of the anaesthetic gas, inevitably some leaks out into the room to be inhaled by staff members. Over the course of the day, on a high-volume, high-turnover list, we have probably inhaled more gas than we realise, albeit at very much sub-anaesthetic concentrations.[9] Staff starting work in paediatric practice are naïve to the effects of breathing the

---

8 Although we seem to manage to work our way around this when siting labour epidurals in wiggling parturients.

9 I will reassure the reader that the anaesthetists, nurses and surgeons are not, in fact, anaesthetised when operating. One has to breathe very high concentrations of the gases continuously to actually enter a state of anaesthesia. The odd accidental whiff has no acutely impairing effect.

low concentrations of gas. I note the student nurse in the room looking a bit taken aback.

The first few weeks anaesthetising children leaves one incapacitated by the time they arrive home. The frequent inhalation of the tiny concentrations of gas accumulates over the course of the day. At the start, barely able to cycle home, I would land on the sofa and fall into a deep slumber by 7 p.m. This effect wears off quickly and we seem to tolerate this persistent minuscule dose of gas. However, I feel like the month off between London and Dublin has left me completely naïve again. I suffer that familiar, but long-forgotten feeling, of complete exhaustion as I arrive home. It is impossible to fight the sofa snooze. I waken an hour later with my jacket still on. Still, better than in the operating theatre, I suppose.

9 – The Surgeon, the Stitch and the Wardrobe

An operation can't start without an anaesthetist, for obvious reasons. You could try, but you may get a swift puck in the nose if you took a scalpel to the abdomen of an awake patient. But it is possible to get to an advanced stage of a procedure without a consultant surgeon. The rest of the team can get to work. The anaesthetist and anaesthetic nurse can knock the patient out in the anaesthetic room. The healthcare assistant will bring the parents out of the theatre department. The porters come and help us transfer the child into the operating theatre. The theatre nurses help us position the child on the operating table and attach all the monitoring. The scrub nurses get the sterile drapes and instruments prepared. The surgical trainee arrives for our last safety check before sterilising the patient's skin and positioning the drapes. Senior surgical registrars will get started on the operation themselves. Only at this point do we need the consultant surgeon.

'Has anyone seen the surgeon?'

'No. He called earlier to say he was ready and to put the child to sleep.'

'That was 25 minutes ago – did you call him again?'

'Yes.'

'And?'

'No answer.'

I wish I knew where they went. I feel like I'm missing out. I picture some little oasis accessed via a secret door at the back of operating theatre 9¾, which only permits entry if you can tie an Aberdeen knot in under 0.5 seconds.[10] I imagine you enter by gliding through the gap in the wardrobe that houses the stock of urinary catheters and colostomy bags. You arrive to be warmly greeted by all your surgical colleagues, alive and dead. You sit on comfortable bean bags, drink fancy coffee, eat muffins and watch re-runs of your favourite operations on TV. Crucially, there's no phone reception and rule number one is never to tell a soul that you are in surgical Narnia. Bliss.

We waited 45 minutes this afternoon in theatre with no sign of our surgeon. The child was anaesthetised, the nurses scrubbed and ready, the surgical registrar as bemused as we were. Out of nowhere the surgeon reappeared from Narnia, with a smile, but no explanation, a urinary catheter and colostomy bag stuck to his back. On this occasion, seeing as we were marching through our list at a mighty rate anyway, I could not get frustrated. We would finish on time even if the surgeon chose to stay in Narnia for a second Swedish massage. Other times, though, lulls in the day can be frustrating, especially for anaesthetists and nurses. We can be in theatre up to an hour after the surgeons are gone, ensuring that the patients are awake and suitable for discharge to the wards – meaning that they're following commands, pain is under control and vital signs

---

10 I don't know what an Aberdeen knot is, but it's the only knot name I can remember from my one and only surgical skills course as an intern.

ok. But, there is no point ever getting annoyed about things you can't control. And until we get the surgical tracking devices working properly or robotic scrub suits, we'll be waiting for the elusive surgeons to return from their daily dip in Narnia's thermal saltwater baths.

10 – Heartbroken

Today is my first taste back in my specialist field, broken hearts.

(A quick, basic tutorial on the 'normal' heart. The heart is a fairly simple arrangement of four chambers and four valves, resulting in two pumps. It is an incredibly powerful muscle. Its function is probably the most basic, yet fundamental, of all the organ systems: to relentlessly squeeze blood around the body in order to move oxygen from the lungs to every single living cell in the body. It almost seems impossible to think that this pump can run, mostly problem free, from our very early days as an embryo until the day we die.)

Congenital heart disease is bizarre. Some of the abnormal arrangements developing hearts manage to get themselves into in utero resemble some sort of Frankenstein heart patched together with Play-Doh, willy-nilly, by some toddler with a limited attention span. Although some are fatal, others that would appear to be unable to support life can, and do, manage to survive for days, weeks or even years with no intervention. Blood goes in the wrong direction, whole valves or chambers of the heart are missing, some babies turn blue – it goes against everything you were taught about how the heart works. In fact, I can barely remember being taught anything about congenital heart disease in medical school as it was too niche and probably too complex for undergraduates.

While kids can survive with congenital heart disease for a period of time without treatment, their development and ability to live a normal childhood can be very limited. These days, all but the most devastating anatomical heart arrangements are amenable to some intervention, which isn't always curative. Treatments include medications, surgery or sometimes interventional cardiac catheter procedures performed by a cardiologist. Think along the lines of the angiogram your grandad had after his heart attack, but for kids. Naturally, they all require general anaesthesia, in contrast to adults.

It takes many years to understand the different pathologies and speak the acronym-heavy congenital cardiac language: HLHS, VSD, MAPCA, VAD, TOF. *This baby has a double-outlet right ventricle, Fallot-type, severe pulmonary stenosis, hypoplastic pulmonary arteries with at least two major aortopulmonary collateral arteries.* It might as well be Mandarin. At the beginning, I would draw a rudimentary heart and then start annotating it with an 'X' and arrows and scribbles to delineate what was actually going on. It's not something that is picked up in a week. It is complicated and one of those subjects that, no matter how many times it is explained to you, you need to sit down and find the part of it that simply 'clicks' the rest of it into place for your style of learning. As you might imagine, it can be tough on trainees, but I love to teach the physiology of this subject. It gets me strangely jittery and excitable. Mostly so I can save someone a whole lot of time trying to figure out a topic on their own, having spent a lot of time banging my own head on the desk trying to grasp it.

Our high-risk case today was in a child with severe pulmonary hypertension. Pulmonary hypertension is essentially high blood pressure in the lungs. The powerful left ventricle can pump blood into the arteries of someone with the more common high blood pressure (hypertension) you would be familiar with. But the weaker right ventricle, which pumps blood to the lungs, is not suited for pumping against high pressure (the pressure in the lungs is much lower usually). If you develop pulmonary hypertension, your right ventricle can easily fail. This makes sufferers some of the highest risk patients for anaesthesia. The cardiologists are performing a pulmonary vascular resistance (PVR) study to assess the severity of a child's pulmonary hypertension. I see the blood drain out of the registrar's face when I explain the risks involved. But like everything in anaesthesia, we have a contingency plan should the shit hit the fan. After inspecting today's fan, however, we found no evidence of excrement, much to the relief of my bamboozled registrar.

12 – Fifteen Minutes, Tops

As soon as you have 'CONSULTANT' branded on your hospital ID badge, some attitudes towards you change. As a trainee, consultants from other specialties would often seem intimidating and there was rarely any banter or chit-chat with them. Their conversation was reserved for your superior anaesthesia overlord. But since I have crossed that threshold and joined the club, I have felt welcomed and my new consultant colleagues seem eager to hear about my training journey and particularly the time I have spent abroad. Some have also completed fellowships in Great Ormond Street Hospital and naturally there is an acceptance for 'alumni' of the same institution. The conversation rapidly moves to tales of yore and I am peppered with enquiries about whether 'such-and-such' is still working there. 'Do they still do that?' 'How many cases do they perform now?' 'He was a bit of a bollocks, the nurses hated him. So did I, to be honest.' Everyone is fascinated by how things are done in other hospitals. The fascination is twofold. Firstly, people are eager to hear if you have come across any new ideas or if there are any techniques that you have honed abroad. Secondly, and more honestly, people are more eager to hear about how we, at this hospital, are the best at whatever it may be. 'I knew we were better than them at that.'

After we collectively decide that our hospital is the best in the world and give ourselves a pat on the back, we must embark on the day's work. There is healthy scepticism that goes back and forth between surgeon and anaesthetist. Neither truly 100 per cent trusts what the other is saying. I know surgeons are incapable of predicting how long an operation will take. Fact. Similarly, I know surgeons don't believe us when we say how long it will take to prepare a patient for theatre. If only we could all just be honest with each other. *Sigh*. The nightmare for the anaesthetist is when a surgeon announces that the operation will be 'a quick 15-minute job'. This means they will be operating until the next solar eclipse.[11] What is generally not considered is the time it takes to wake the previous patient, retrieve the next patient up from the ward, actually anaesthetise the next patient, run through all the safety checks, position the patient, drape the patient, do the crossword, file your tax return, switch off the immersion … all before the surgery can begin. Nothing is ever *just* 15 minutes. But the surgical consultant today is a pro. He puts the pro in professor. Forty years of experience give him a unique ability to be entirely realistic about his surgical prowess. He plans his list with such accuracy that we finish with about two minutes to spare in our allotted theatre time. It's 16.58, the sweet spot. Theatre management give us a round of applause and a guard of honour as we vacate the theatre.

15 – A Dicky Heart

When the surgeon or medical consultant calls you the day before a list to discuss a patient, you know it must be serious. Quite often, anaesthetists only meet the patients on the operating list on the morning of surgery, so receiving a 'pre-warning' in advance suggests that we may have a complicated patient or a new surgical procedure to contend with.

Anaesthetists, in jest, give surgeons (particularly orthopaedic surgeons) a hard time about their basic medical knowledge. They're

---

11 According to surgeons, the anaesthetist's equivalent of a surgeon's 'quick 15-minute job' is 'I'm just going to do a quick regional block'.

easy targets; you just have to stand outside an orthopaedic theatre to confirm that it sounds more like a woodwork classroom than a place of delicate, intricate surgery. A surgeon's diagnosis of common medical problems can include: 'a dicky heart', 'dodgy lungs' or the elusive 'infection of some sort'. If the surgeon is taking the time to call you, the patient must be at death's door. Frankly, we are delighted to be forewarned about challenging cases in order to prepare accordingly. Last night it was a cardiologist calling me, concerned about one of their patients that I would be anaesthetising today. If a cardiologist is concerned then I really need to sit up and listen.

The cardiologist is concerned about a child with a Fontan circulation. This is at the advanced end of congenital heart disease and not something that most anaesthetists will ever see, unless of course you work in a paediatric cardiac centre. The Fontan operation is the final palliative (not curative) operation for children born with the devastating diagnosis of hypoplastic left heart syndrome (HLHS), with which they effectively only have one major pumping chamber (ventricle) in their heart,[12] and it's not the strong one. There is no cure for HLHS but several operations are performed to make the heart configuration they have fractionally more efficient. When you reach the Fontan stage, some patients do well and survive to adolescence or young adulthood, but ultimately a heart transplant is the only long-term strategy, the Catch-22 being that many are too unwell for a successful transplant. Our little patient, Sarah, has what is described as a 'failing Fontan'. Her system is already working so inefficiently that a transplant is probably her only hope of long-term survival, but her chances of receiving one are minute. Her oxygen saturations are 75 per cent, where they should be about 95 per cent in a well-functioning

12 The Fontan circulation is also the end-point for some other very complex congenital heart diseases.

Fontan circulation (or 100 per cent in someone with a healthy heart). This is a high-risk anaesthetic.

Today I am covering the MRI machine. Unlike adults, it will come as no surprise that a tiny child will not lie perfectly still inside a cold, tubular coffin listening to what sounds like rabid bleating goats on a background of intermittent distorted alien voices crackling through the intercom. You would be forgiven for thinking you were on a one-way ticket to Mars. Thus, most children under the age of eight or so receive a general anaesthetic for their MRI scan. The scanner is usually in a remote location from the operating theatre complex. Like many things, there is safety in numbers and high-risk procedures of any kind are best done where there are many people around in case of emergency. So ideally, high-risk children who require a general anaesthetic would be best anaesthetised during the day, on a planned list, in the main theatre complex. 'Remote anaesthesia' is regularly flagged in our training as a place where bad things could potentially happen. Even being a three-minute walk away from theatre can feel as remote as being in the middle of the Sahara Desert, though infection control would likely rule this out anyway. One must be extra-cautious when preparing for high-risk cases in an environment 'remote' from theatre.

Sarah needs an MRI scan to evaluate a large collection of fluid she has in her chest. Cases like this are challenging and complex. Anaesthetists inexperienced in paediatric cardiac anaesthesia would never anaesthetise this child, as too many things could go wrong. But doing cases like this is what makes paediatric practice so rewarding. Sometimes you have to step to the very edge of your comfort zones to do what is right by the patient. I take some time to discuss the particular physiological concepts unique to a Fontan circulation with my registrar. This involves drawing a diagram of the heart not worthy of little Sarah's best crayon work.

Despite the risk, there is no undue excitement with her in the MRI machine. Everything goes smoothly. In anaesthesia, no unexpected excitement usually means you've done a good job. A boring anaesthetic is a safe one.

17 – 'No' Is a Complete Sentence

My consultant surgical colleague today clearly doesn't have the keys to Narnia yet. Ever present and ready to operate, together we cruise through our six cases and are finished by 3.30 p.m. Despite being excited by the prospect of an early departure home, I tell myself it's always a team effort and check in on my anaesthetic colleagues to see if I can help to keep their operating lists ticking over.

Enthusiasm goes a long way in medicine. As a student, if you hung around with a specialist registrar late into the day, you would be rewarded with the chance to scrub and assist in theatre or get an impromptu tutorial with some crucial pearls of wisdom for exams. As a trainee anaesthetist, being seen as eager to work and willing to stay late occasionally ultimately led to the consultants having more trust in you, and your being rewarded with more independence. Ideally, this trait should continue throughout one's career in medicine, but it can be readily forgotten. Enthusiasm is one thing, but being a 'Yes' man is another. I'm the new consultant and it appears that I'm becoming overly agreeable.

'Can we start this major operation late in the day?'

'Yes.'

'Will you cover me this afternoon?'

'Yes.'

'Will you raise €10 million for a new intensive care unit?'

'Yes.'

'Will you collect my children from school?'

'Yes.'

'Please can you take my mother-in-law to the opera on Saturday?'

'My pleasure!'

But it isn't a fault, it's a desire to be welcomed and become part of the team. It's so common that the same advice was thrust upon me by multiple people before I started – don't be afraid to say 'No'. This was often followed by, 'Your clinical work is most important at the beginning, so don't take on extra tasks or roles.' Let's be honest: it's solid advice, but it's going out the window as I'm on bloody probation for the first year so I am willing and ready to do whatever it takes to stay on the team.[13]

I agree to take over the final case on an operating list for a colleague who needs to leave early for family reasons. It's not a big deal as the operation appears to be winding up and should be done in 30 minutes. No problem. Fast forward to three hours later, the surgery is well finished but I'm the only anaesthetist left in the operating department. The baby is in recovery but not well enough to be discharged to the wards. I'm racking my brains as to why the baby I was left with has a heart rate of 180 (fast, even for a baby). After cursing myself for being helpful, I get to the bottom of the problem, eventually. I get home just after 8 p.m. It's part of my initiation onto the team.

The advice I received the next morning was, 'Next time, tell them to fuck off.'

22 – Jelly Baby

Every day, one consultant from each specialty is designated as the 'on-call' person. For us, this means anaesthetising any children that need emergency surgery. After hours, when everyone else goes home, you are the sole anaesthetist available to provide this service. Today

---

13 All new consultant posts in Ireland have a hefty one-year probationary period, just so they can be sure you're not the next Harold Shipman. They'd like to nip that one in the bud early. It is proving a sticking point in my mortgage applications. My probation that is, not me being a mass murderer.

is a big day. It is my first day as the 'on-call' anaesthetist for the hospital. Unsurprisingly, this is where you really feel most vulnerable as a new consultant. All your helpful and supportive colleagues are tucked up in their beds and not in the theatre next door where they would normally be available for advice. Towards the end of the normal working day, it is with great relief that I hear my colleagues reminiscing of their first nights on call and many of them quietly offer their ear on the end of the phone should I need advice overnight. Some even offer to come in if I really need help. I am most thankful for this. *One pair of underpants should do for the night.*

It is a double hit as today is also my first day anaesthetising children for open cardiac surgery since I started. Having spent all my time on fellowship in London working with children with congenital heart disease, the cases listed don't faze me, and I'm skipping on the way into work. Due to the way the roster falls, I will always work with the same cardiac surgeon, so it is an opportunity to build a good working relationship with both the surgeon and the perfusionists.[14] Three-way communication between us is crucial in this type of surgery.

We have two cases today. Our first patient is a baby who has Trisomy 21 (Down's syndrome).[15] Many children with Trisomy 21 have cardiac abnormalities, and this little baby has a complete atrio-ventricular septal defect (CAVSD). This is rare in the general population, but really quite common in those with Trisomy 21 and it almost always requires surgery. We operate on lots of complex, neonatal heart defects, with CAVSD being one of the more common. Children with congenital heart disease are usually diagnosed in the

---

14 Perfusionists are clinical scientists responsible for the operation of the cardio-pulmonary bypass machine, to support the patient when their heart and lungs are stopped during open heart surgery.

15 Kids with Down's syndrome have three copies of chromosome 21 where most people have two. Trisomy means 'three chromosomes'.

antenatal period. Parents of children with congenital heart disease are thoroughly counselled on treatment options and long-term outcomes for whatever specific congenital heart defect we are presented with. Our expert cardiologists and cardiac surgeons only make recommendations.

We finish our two cases by 8 p.m. At this stage, I have to turn my attention to any emergency surgeries that remain pending. My colleagues have cleared almost all the emergencies during the day and we are left with an appendicectomy to perform.[16] I allow my registrar some independence and I let him get on with it while I remain in the theatre office within earshot.

Later, as I prepare to leave, I receive a call from a medical consultant who has another child with Trisomy 21 on the ward. The medical team have been struggling to gain IV access for almost eight hours. Anaesthetists are seen as the 'experts' in venous access. Whether this is justified or not is debatable. Patients arrive back from the operating theatre to the wards with cannulas bigger than other doctors ever knew existed. This is jaw-dropping to some, as they may have struggled to insert even the smallest IV on the ward pre-operatively. The secret here is that it's quite easy to cannulate a perfectly still target and not so easy to cannulate a wriggling, hysterical baby. Our anaesthetic drugs also dilate the veins somewhat and we have ultrasound machines to find elusive veins. The experts are really the IV nurses who work on the wards. But, occasionally, they fail too. The last solution, and one we don't take lightly, is to bring the baby to the operating theatre. Here I can anaesthetise the baby

---

16 Before working in the operating theatre, the word 'emergency' would always result in visions of CPR, panic and blood from watching chaotic resuscitations on *ER* or other medical television dramas. When we say 'emergency', it is rarely a case of literally rushing someone to theatre and the surgeon operating in his Bermuda shorts with the car still running in the car park. 'Urgent' is probably a better word – the surgery needs to be done soon, usually within 24 hours. There are occasionally 'true emergencies' that are time sensitive and must be done ASAP.

to keep them still and take my time with an ultrasound machine to scan the limbs, neck and groins for suitable veins.

The ultrasound machine requires a gel to transmit the ultrasound waves that the technology is based on. After using so much lubrication to scan the baby all over for a suitable vein, they're as slick as a wet fish. Eventually I settle on a central line placed in the femoral vein, in the baby's groin. It's late and I'm tired, but it is safer and better for the baby's care to get this done tonight, I wouldn't like to leave the medical team stuck and the baby needs intravenous antibiotics. It's 1 a.m. by the time I leave the hospital.

With no more calls overnight, I am safe in the knowledge that I have completed my first night on call as a consultant. Another stepping-stone. It feels like I've properly started now.

24 – This Is Awkward

Everyone graduates from medicine with the same basic medical knowledge, more or less. But very quickly thereafter, individuals move rapidly into their chosen specialties. There is some crossover of knowledge, but let's be honest, a few years into training and I would not expect a geriatrician to be able to recall a child's vaccination schedule or expect an orthopaedic surgeon to list the causes of pre-term labour. And you certainly wouldn't want me operating on you.

It doesn't happen very often, but it will happen to every anaesthetist at least once in their careers: the opportunity to anaesthetise a fellow doctor or, worse, a fellow doctor's child. The prospect of this is daunting for a number of reasons – you expect them to quiz you about the minutiae of your specialty, you expect them to not trust anyone unless they are a world-leading expert in their field and, personally, I expect them to look at me with suspicion, as I don't look particularly distinguished; the facial hair goes some ways to hiding the teenager's face beneath. On the plus side, you expect fellow doctors to listen intently to everything you're saying and have a better understanding of risk and complications than your average patient. Inevitably, all these worries are unfounded as, like I said, no one remembers anything they learned about anaesthesia in medical school. It seems we can get away with it. Other doctors don't seem to have a clue what we do. Fellow doctors just appear to trust anaesthetists wholly and completely, and very rarely have any questions to ask. I'm not sure where this stems from. Perhaps they witnessed an anaesthetist managing a complex patient of theirs in the ICU or perhaps, more simply, they acknowledge that there is no surgery without anaesthesia, so they have no choice but to trust us. Fellow medic or not, they still have to sit and listen to my little explanatory speech, so I can make sure they take in the same information I would give to any parent.

In London, I very nearly had to anaesthetise my boss's child for an appendicectomy – the consultant who hired me, the one whom I worked alongside every day, the one who would write my reference for any future job applications. Suddenly, a very simple anaesthetic looked somewhat challenging. *Let's get the 'difficult airway' trolley ready. I think we'll need 17 IV cannulas. Let's ring intensive care and ask for a post-op bed.* As the senior fellow on call in the evening, with everyone else (including the consultants) gone home, I had the final word regarding the order in which we would perform the remaining emergency operations. I gulped as I walked up the stairs to explain to my own boss that her child would have to wait as there was a more urgent case to be done first. She glared straight through me.[17] As a courtesy, I let the consultant on call know the situation and I got a very swift reply: 'Don't worry, I'll come in and do that case!' My shift ended as they were making their way to theatre later in the evening. I still got my reference.

---

17 Later, on full explanation, she acknowledged that the tiny, semi-conscious baby requiring a ventriculo-peritoneal shunt (a tube that passes from the ventricles in the brain under the skin to the abdomen) probably did qualify to be operated on before her kid.

Today I had to anaesthetise a fellow consultant's child so that they could fix a broken arm. The consultant in question practised a specialty quite remote from anaesthesia. Initially, I played it safe, I talked medically, on what I hoped was common ground. I was only moments into my speech about the safety of anaesthesia in young children based on the most recent research when I saw his eyes begin to glaze. It appeared as if he was trying to spell supercalifragilisticexpialidocious backwards. He wasn't listening to a word I was saying. *Tone it down.* I defaulted to my layman's explanation of anaesthesia, to which he appeared much more receptive; I had to remind myself, he's a parent first and foremost. Satisfied with my credentials, we got under way.

26 – Verra Smol Baybees

When I see the operating list today, I get both nervous and excited. My thoughts rush back to my challenging case in my first week when I got slightly burned by inexperience. I learned so much during that one case, and having dissected it with some senior colleagues, I had a fully formulated plan in my head on what I would do for the next similar case.

Surgery in tiny preemies is relatively rare, so today's case is my first opportunity to chase away the ghosts of the previous case. It's not exactly the same, but close enough. Ciaran is an *ex-prem* and suffers from many of the chronic complications of prematurity: he is on oxygen all the time; he has some support with his ventilation; he has already had one emergency surgery for a perforated bowel and has a stoma.[18] He cannot take any food orally, only via a long-

---

18 A stoma is where part of the bowel is externalised to allow faeces to drain into a bag attached to the skin. It can be used as an end point of surgery or be a temporary measure to allow the bowel to heal following an emergency bowel operation. (I know there are other types of stoma, surgeons – don't judge me.)

term IV line – this is called total parenteral nutrition or TPN for short. It provides him with calories, but sometimes not as much as traditional baby food. He is five months old now but weighs only a feeble 3.2 kg, which is below the average weight of a healthy baby born at term. A healthy five-month-old would be over the 6 kg mark. It doesn't seem like much of a difference, but it really is. The smaller the baby, the trickier the technical side of surgery and anaesthesia. But he is doing well enough to come to us today to reverse his stoma and sew his healthy bowel back together again.

An old technique I was taught and practised regularly when playing high-level, competitive hockey was 'visualisation'. In the preparation for a match I would picture the first pass, picture the first tackle, picture the first sprint. You build a mental picture of what it will feel like to perform the first successful small tasks in the game. Visualise it. Do the basic things well and the rest will follow. All morning I find myself, unknowingly (and as corny as it sounds), visualising each step I will carry out for this anaesthetic to be successful. But it is a valuable exercise to stave off any anxiety around the case.

The major issue for this ex-prem is not his size, but his lungs. Premature lungs are not healthy. They can be extremely stiff, scarred and poor at performing the primary basic task of the lungs, which is transferring oxygen from the air into the bloodstream. The metabolic rate of a baby is extremely high, compared to an adult, so they use a lot of oxygen and their lungs don't store much in reserve. We can measure oxygen levels using an oxygen saturation monitor ('sats' monitor) which will be familiar to anyone who has been in a hospital or had an operation. Normal saturations are 100 per cent if you are breathing air, of which 21 per cent is pure oxygen.

After filling an adult's lungs with extra oxygen before rendering them apnoeic (unable to breathe) at the start of an anaesthetic, you will have several minutes before their normal oxygen saturations of 100 per cent started to drop to 99 per cent ... 98 per cent ... 97 per cent … We call this 'desaturation'. This relatively slow rate of desaturation is due to their large reserve and lower metabolic rate. If you do the same with a healthy baby, you might have 15–20 seconds before they begin to desaturate. Their lungs can't store as much oxygen, and they churn through whatever oxygen is available very quickly. Consider an ex-prem with diseased, stiff lungs and you're talking almost immediate desaturation when they stop breathing, or sometimes their saturations don't even get above 90 per cent with additional oxygen. It is like paddling along a slow river and then suddenly crashing over Niagara Falls.

When a patient stops breathing at the start of a general anaesthetic, anaesthetists take over. We use either a hand-operated inflatable bag or a mechanical ventilator to blow air into the lungs. The term we would use is 'ventilation'. We 'ventilate' the patient's lungs. To facilitate ventilation, we place an endotracheal tube (ETT) via the nose or mouth into the trachea, the tunnel that runs into the lungs. Avoiding desaturation is one of the primary goals of the anaesthetist because prolonged low oxygen levels can lead to cardiac arrest. The effervescent, high pitched *pip … pip … pip … pip* that sounds in unison with the heartbeat when saturations are over 97 per cent are music to the anaesthetist's ears. As the saturations drop, the tone grumbles down to a horrifying *dum … dummmmm … mmmmm … ghhhhhhh*. Enough to make any anaesthetist have a stroke.[19]

I am telling you this, not only for educational purposes but, as you might have expected, the saturations of today's ex-prem briefly sounded like the grim reaper was in the operating room, a hand on my shoulder, his cold breath on my neck and gently whispering into my ear *dum … dummmmm … mmmmm … ghhhhhhh*. Our start-

---

19 I have often thought that once the saturations drop below 70 per cent, we should hear some calming or motivation music instead, just to settle our own heart rates. Maybe 'Daddy Cool' or 'Eye of the Tiger'.

ing point with Ciaran was saturations of 92 per cent and he was already receiving supplemental oxygen pre-operatively. Difficult and challenging. Initially everything was A-OK, as my more junior colleague had skilfully and successfully intubated the baby with an oral tube. With this endo-tracheal tube safely in position, we opted to change it for a nasal tube, which is a more comfortable position if the ETT is to be in place for several days in the PICU, where he would be going post-operatively. This is a more advanced manoeuvre and can be tricky in small babies because, well, they're verra smol.

Fully confident that my junior colleague was capable of performing this technique and with everything looking well, I let him press on. He has a look into the back of the mouth with a laryngoscope.[20] Having already threaded the nasal tube through the nose and into the back of the throat, he can see it sitting next to the oral tube which is through the vocal cords and sitting neatly in the trachea, where it belongs. This is perfect. As you can imagine, having two silicone tubes, a laryngoscope and a forceps (used to pick up the nasal tube and direct it through the vocal cords) all within the throat of a tiny baby doesn't leave a whole lot of room to manoeuvre. The next step is to remove the oral tube out from the vocal cords to allow space for the nasal tube to pass into the trachea. Great. Saturations 94 per cent. Now, some fumbling. 'Everything ok?' More fumbling. Saturations 89 per cent. 'Can you advance the tube?' No reply. Saturations 83 per cent. 'Tell me what you see?' Saturations 78 per cent. 'You need to pass the tube or come out!' Saturations 72 per cent. 'I can't see anything, I've lost my view of the trachea.' Nightmare. Saturations 54 per cent. *Dum … dum … mmmm …*

---

20 A laryngoscope is the device we use to get a clear view of the vocal cords, the gates to the trachea. The 'larynx' being the cartilaginous structure you can feel in the front of your neck (the Adam's apple). It looks a bit like a gynaecological speculum, but I am yet to try using it to visualise the cervix.

At this point I take over control and revert to basic ventilation techniques – using a mask and a bag to blow highly concentrated oxygen into the baby's lungs. Saturations 70 per cent. The lungs are so stiff. Even a brief spell without ventilation and it's now very difficult to get air to move into the lungs. With each squeeze of the bag, the air prefers to head down into the stomach where there is less resistance. A big distended belly doesn't help the situation. The air in the stomach increases the pressure in the abdomen, which in turn increases the pressure in the thorax, making successfully ventilating the lungs even harder. It's a vicious circle. Saturations 60 per cent. I rapidly ask the nurses to get me an endotracheal tube so I can place an oral tube back in. Saturations 55 per cent. There is blood in the back of the mouth now from the trauma of the previous attempts. I can't see anything. Saturations 48 per cent. The heart rate now dropping. We're heading for cardiac arrest.

'Press the emergency bell!' This alerts the entire operating theatre of an emergency in need of immediate assistance. I look again and through the blood I can see a tiny opening through what might be the vocal cords. I push the tube down. Saturations 40 per cent. *Dum … dummmmm … mmmmm … ghhhhhhh.* I think I'm in. I squeeze the bag. The lungs aren't moving. I'm certain the tube is in the trachea. I squeeze harder. Finally, some movement. The other signs of a successfully placed ETT appear. Saturations 60 per cent. The tube is definitely in. Saturations 80 per cent. The doors of the operating theatre burst open – help has arrived. Saturations 90 per cent. The first consultant to arrive asks if all is ok. 'Oh, just a bit of trouble intubating,' I answer, casually. Saturations 97 per cent *pip … pip … pip … pip.* Heart rate normal. Another colleague interjects, 'Is that Ciaran? I anaesthetised him for a procedure last week – he was a nightmare.'

That entire scenario probably lasted less than 30 seconds. It is a strange sensation when faced with these critical scenarios. Over the course of training, you face so many of them. Everything slows down, a second feels like a minute, it feels like you have time to rectify the situation. My dad used to point out great footballers who never seemed to look rushed on the ball. They *always* had time. He would note that they were so aware of their surroundings and their first touch was so good that they could create time and space. They knew what they were going to do with the ball before they got it. While I am no Cesc Fàbregas, I can honestly say that I never feel stressed when I am in the throes of a full-blown crisis. I just can't be, as I am the one that needs to fix the problem. You need situational awareness and you know, automatically, what needs to be done if a trainee or anyone else is struggling. With time and practice, you know that your skills are good enough for you to intervene and rectify a situation quickly (your 'first touch'). But always, afterwards, when the crisis is sorted, you become acutely aware of your own heart rate. The thud in your head as your raised blood pressure pounds your temples. The adrenalin letting its presence be felt.

The emergency bells go off in a paediatric operating theatre at least once or twice a week. In comparison, I can probably count on one hand how many times this happened in all my experience in adult hospitals. But this is why I love paediatric anaesthesia – because it is hard. Despite this 30 seconds of coronary-squeezing and bowel-loosening hysteria, the rest of the procedure was a joy and we were extremely pleased with how we managed this verra smol ex-prem.

30 – Snowflakes

When the snowflakey millennials over in the Google and Facebook offices are given the day off because the weather is a little bit cold, it makes me wonder how we, in frontline healthcare, are expected to trudge through whatever seasonal fiasco is thrown in our wake. The hospital is always expected to function as normal, for emergencies at the very least. These are inevitable. I accept these impassable days don't happen too frequently, but the effort made by frontline medical staff is often underappreciated.

Despite snow falling last night, my registrar had attempted a cross-country drive to get to work this morning. I got a text from him late last night to inform me, dejectedly, that he had been forced to turn his car around when driving from Cork to Dublin. I pictured him battening down the hatches on the side of the motorway, cursing the fact that he would miss a day's work. With the engine still running to keep the heat up and blowing the cold from his hands, he sent one last desperate text to work to say, 'Sorry, I have let you down,' his frozen corpse erected on the side of the M7 for ever more.

So, I resigned myself to a day working solo. I considered how this would affect the working day. Similar weather in London last year had meant that many patients couldn't get to the hospital for scheduled surgery; we all somehow managed to trudge in (after various travel calamities) only to be sent home again, as there were very few patients who had braved the elements. I was somewhat concerned that tomorrow would be a repeat of that wasteful day.[21]

As I sat at home watching the snow actually stick to the ground, I groaned. I wondered if I would make it in to provide anaesthesia for the ten children on the list for endoscopies and colonoscopies. There's a real treat for a kid on a snow day; as all your pals gather in the local park to throw snowballs at each other and get their tongues stuck to lampposts, you'd be at home glued to the toilet seat with unrelenting diarrhoea as a result of the laxatives required to get those bowels ready for the colonoscopy you didn't even ask

---

21 I have to say it was wasteful as we didn't get any work done. But seeing as I got a hot chocolate and made a partial snowman in Regent's Park, it was personally very productive.

for. To top that off, there would be no warm bowl of soup to heat up those cold bones – you're fasting. In the morning, you will be woken, against your will, at an absurdly early hour to sit in snail-like snowy traffic with a parent cursing their fellow drivers. Finally, the reward for this perseverance? A camera up your arse.

As usual, the snow didn't quite get thick enough to cause mass panic and services were uninterrupted, much to my disappointment.

31 – We Do Not Negotiate with Terrorists

It is hard to predict how a child will react when they arrive to be anaesthetised. Although I may act like one sometimes, I have been reminded that I am not a child and thus can't relate to how they must feel in a hospital. I was never anaesthetised as a child either, so I have no point of reference. But I can imagine what it is like to have a stranger tell you you're going to be gassed, thrust a mask into your face and have your parents, the ones you trust the most, endorsing the assault.

You have to take different tactics with different age groups. Small babies, less than six months of age, are easy; they don't know what's happening, and they don't fight. It's the parents who are most distraught with this age group, and there have been occasions when parents have refused to leave the operating theatre, which is not an ideal or safe situation when you are trying to manage the airway of a little baby. It's understandable in the building apprehension of a small baby having surgery, which is hugely upsetting for parents.

Ages one to three years are generally a nightmare. You cannot reason with a terrorist. They have no comprehension, only mistrust. The 'hugs' from Mummy and Daddy are a gentler form of restraint than the Hannibal Lector-style approach that would be more effective, but sadly unethical. There are *always* tears. *Always*. First the child cries as this process is against their unflappable wishes. Then the parent cries as they have temporarily broken the bond of trust (maybe for the first time) with their little one. Then the anaesthetist cries. You have to be there to witness it, but as the toddler starts to fall asleep, there are inevitably a few glances from the child up to the monster holding the mask. The look of 'why are you doing this to me?' is utterly heart-breaking.

Ages four to eight can go either way. Some are so keen to try the mask that they essentially anaesthetise themselves. This is not linked to future drug abuse. Others are a bit coy but can be talked around with a bit of parental assistance. The third group in this cohort can just flat refuse – either through anxiety or strong-mindedness. They comprehend the situation, they have a sense of agency and they just know this is a game that they don't want to play. *Sorry, doctor, would you mind pissing off? I'm watching my iPad and there is no way I'm letting you get in the way of today's rendition of* Frozen. This is a group that can benefit from a premedication, which is usually an oral medication aimed at getting the kid to chill out a little bit.

Once the kids get to nine or so, I offer them the choice of either the mask or an IV. Over 12, you're getting an IV, full stop. The heavier you become, the longer it takes you to fall unconscious using the mask and gas. The intravenous route is a lot faster by this stage. You have to be careful, though, how much choice you give a kid. I can appreciate my fellow consultants and nursing staff who have kids of their own and are used to dealing with those who want to be in control of everything. For example:

Kid: 'If you think I'm having surgery today well then you can forget it.' (Cue tears/tantrum – delete as appropriate.)

Helpful parent/experienced anaesthetist or surgeon: 'Well, actually, you're not old enough to make that decision. We have decided you need this operation so that's not negotiable, but we will give you some choice on how it happens.'

To be fair to the child, their fear is usually born out of a previous bad experience or, simply, the unknown – although some are just being dicks to their parents.

Today we had a rollercoaster of a ride trying to coax a young pre-teen patient into going to sleep. She was a healthy child, but had a previous traumatic experience with anaesthesia about two years ago. You can meet a child pre-operatively on the ward before surgery, explain your role and come away from the discussion with the impression that the child is on board with everything and there-fore things will go smoothly. But on arrival to the anaesthetic room, you would be forgiven for thinking ISIS has sent their top cadet as a replacement. Today the initial plan was to attempt an IV (child's choice), then we weren't, then there was hyperventilation, then screaming at Dad, then we tried the mask, blind panic, then walk-ing out of the anaesthetic room, then crying, then back to the IV, no wait, back to the mask … cue tantrum, then finally the child put herself to sleep with the mask. The process took nearly 40 minutes – a long time when you're trying to run a smooth, timely theatre list.

It can be so hard to predict this kind of behaviour, and some-times it's entirely unexpected. It's obviously frightening for a child. Unfortunately, we simply don't have the resources for a psycholo-gist to help with every child with anxiety issues who requires general anaesthesia and surgery. For the rare few who do have this luxury, it does have a significant impact. Otherwise, we can just do our best.

36 – Territorial Army

Some things about surgery confuse me, I will admit that. I don't know how many surgical disciplines there are, but to me there seems to be a suspicious amount of crossover in terms of which subspecialty performs which type of surgery. Some straightforward examples: an injury to a bone in the hand might be fixed by an orthopaedic surgery or a plastic surgeon – I don't know how they decide. A woman with stress incontinence might be treated by a gynaecologist or a urologist – I don't know how they decide.

A huge grey area is what happens from the neck up. The following people may operate in this area: an ear, nose and throat (ENT) surgeon, a neurosurgeon, a plastic surgeon, a dental surgeon, a general surgeon, a maxillo-facial surgeon, an oral surgeon, an ophthalmologist, a cranio-facial surgeon or a vascular surgeon. You may even get a distinctly lost orthopaedic surgeon up there. Are they having a laugh? I can't keep up. Why does an ENT surgeon fix your broken nose, but a plastic surgeon will break it and cosmetically straighten it for you? Why does a plastic surgeon repair a cleft palate when the palate is attached to the maxilla – hello *maxillo-facial surgeons?!*

I am working on a maxillo-facial surgery list today and, to be fair, they do some neat and niche surgery beyond removing wisdom teeth. There is a fair bit of reconstructive surgery and this can remind you just how mean kids can be. We are performing a mandibular distraction operation on a teenager with a condition that causes a visible physical malformation to his face. Our patient is being bullied in school. It was the same when I was a teenager, it was the same when my parents were teenagers and it doesn't seem to have changed much now. Teenagers can be horrifically cruel to those who appear superficially different. They can't look past what is on the outside to see the person they are harming on the inside. Surgery to correct these kinds of conditions is not the only reconstructive operation we perform on children who are bullied for their physical appearance; otoplasty is another.

A mandibular distraction is a big operation and it can be painful. The surgeons need to break the jawbone (mandible) to allow distraction plates to be positioned with various screws. The plates get lengthened, essentially with a screwdriver, over the course of several weeks to encourage the mandible to elongate. The goal is to have a more traditional appearance of a jawline and a chin in a more natural position. I hope he does well and, even if the bullies don't stop, he feels more comfortable with himself.

Back to my surgical confusion. At one point in the operation, I counted five surgeons scrubbed in. *Five*. What are they all doing?

37 – A Proper Doctor

As hospital doctors become further and further subspecialised, a similar pattern has emerged in nursing and ancillary staffing also. There are fewer people who can be considered all-rounders. Once upon a time, the same surgeon who operated on your blood vessels would then operate on your thyroid gland, the staff nurse would look after medical, surgical and paediatric patients, the porters would transport patients around the hospital then nip down to the post office to drop off the hospital mail and cleaning staff would work all around the hospital. Now a surgeon can specialise in the smallest part of the body, a nurse can become a specialist in any field and a cleaner can work exclusively in a single operating theatre. Some groups can be quite territorial. I have worked in a hospital where portering staff would refuse to work if anyone so much as moved a patient an inch without their presence as it was 'their job'. Personally, I'm delighted when I'm anaesthetising a patient without a registrar and a skilled nurse places the IV line for me. A little bit of diversity helps.

Today I witnessed the antithesis of subspecialisation: the ultimate doctor. Not only does he operate, he then takes on the role of porter, cleaner, anaesthetic assistant and radiographer. It is equally hilarious, endearing and motivating to see a consultant who is down-to-earth and very much willing to act as a cog in the system as opposed to the hand that turns the wheel. As I put a child off to sleep, he helps the anaesthetic nurse to place the ECG leads and blood-pressure cuff. At one point I head to scrub up before I site an epidural catheter. When I return to the anaesthetic room, the consultant surgeon has turned the child and is holding them in position for me. As his trainees scrub up, he marches out into the corridor to retrieve the x-ray equipment. After the surgery is complete, he picks up the still-anaesthetised child and places them gently on the transfer trolley. As I return from the recovery unit, I see him pushing excess trolleys into the corridor, removing said x-ray equipment and picking up debris left on the floor. Following this, out comes the mop and bucket, and he scrubs the floor well enough to eat your dinner off it – if you like MRSA on your dinner.

Leave your ego at the door; *this* is a proper doctor.

38 – Radioactive Man

The list of things children need general anaesthesia for continues to grow:

Surgery
Intensive care
Dental extractions
MRI and CT scans
Endoscopy
Cannulation
Long car journeys
Bedtime[22]
Wedding ceremonies
The sweets aisle in Tesco
Long-haul flights

---

22 The most common joke from parents after watching their child fall asleep is: 'Can we have some of that for bedtime!' This joke occurs 11 out of 10 times that parents make jokes.

Actually, all flights
Before re-starting *Frozen*. Again.
Before starting *Baby Shark*. Ever.
And now, radiation oncology.

Radiotherapy is a type of cancer treatment that harnesses radiation to reduce the size of tumours, help with cancer pain or to switch off the immune system before a stem cell or bone marrow transplant. It is not particularly common in children but, as always, they have to lie perfectly still for the duration of the treatment. While this service is not available in our hospital, one of us travels to a nearby hospital if there is a child who requires this type of treatment.

Our patient for radiotherapy today is, all things considered, a bright and chirpy little one who is having total-body irradiation for a relapse of leukaemia. This involves two treatments per day (and thus, two general anaesthetics each day) for four days straight. This is in anticipation of a bone marrow or stem cell transplant. The radiotherapy destroys residual cancer cells and tones down the immune system before the new, healthy cells are transplanted. This gruelling week of general anaesthesia would be enough to wear down even the most resilient of kids, but not this one. The main reason, I am convinced, is with the work of a particular porter in the hospital. I was told before arriving just how fantastic this porter was with all the paediatric patients. Over many years working in the hospital, he has established a routine that puts the children at ease when they are on their way for their treatment. He has them assist him in preparing the room, pushing the anaesthetic machine and trolleys around the hospital (with a few staged 'crashes') and even lets them feed the fish. He talks to them about their anaesthetic and tells them how he has had one too.

Come time for the treatment and the general anaesthetic, this little trooper scrambles up on the trolley and even helps put on the monitoring equipment. The 'sleepy medicine' is injected, and that's that. Ancillary staff like our porter here are invaluable to our health system and must be treated with the same respect given to any consultant, board member or service manager. Small things, like his treatment of the kids, are often unseen and unrecognised, but they go a long way to making our job easier.

40 – Bed Roulette

Lack of beds is an infuriating issue in every hospital. It's not fair to patients who are sitting in the emergency department waiting for an inpatient bed, it's not fair for patients who are waiting to be discharged but have no bed in a convalescent home available and it's not fair on patients who have elective surgery cancelled at short notice. This issue tends to be worse in adult hospitals as they have more emergency attendances, more patients who require admission to hospital, convalescence or home-care packages for discharge, and many more patients who require long post-operative stays in the hospital. In a children's hospital, many emergency attendances can be managed without admission, children generally don't need extensive discharge planning and the majority of surgery can be performed on the same day. It is rare for elective children's surgery to be cancelled, but if it is, you have an entire surgical, anaesthesia and nursing team idle, which is an enormous waste of resources. It is rare, but happens at predictable junctures each year.

One type of elective surgery is particularly vulnerable to cancellation for lack of beds: that which requires admission to the PICU post-operatively. It is neither safe nor advisable to carry out surgery where a patient requires PICU admission post-op without establishing if there is a bed available before starting. We don't have many intensive care beds, but we have many patients who require them. As you can imagine, a child who needs this scarce resource is quite likely to be either (a) quite unwell to start with, or (b) having very major surgery, or regularly (c) both. All children having open cardiac surgery require a PICU bed; therefore, the majority of paediatric surgical cases that I have been involved with that have been cancelled have been cardiac surgeries. This is because proceeding with any of these operations is entirely reliant on these beds being available. The nature of cardiac surgery also means that planned cases get bumped for urgent cases, often at short notice. These more urgent cases might be babies who weren't even born when the planned surgical list was drafted. It's therefore only somewhat predictable.

Today is no different. I met two sets of parents of babies with serious cardiac conditions, both requiring surgery, both at home but on several medications. With only one available bed, my mathematical deductions told me that we were one bed short for the two patients requiring surgery today. Whenever I meet any parents on the morning of major surgery, I do my best to manage expectations by explaining that I am not 100 per cent certain we can proceed with surgery until we can confirm that a PICU bed is available.

No matter how much I qualify my statement, it is always crushing for parents to be told their child's surgery is cancelled on any given day. The mental preparation for major surgery is immense, for the parents and the child alike. Being told they must go through it all again tomorrow or the following week or month is hard to take. Many understand, but many vent their frustration, especially if their surgery has been cancelled more than once. The unseen consequences of repeat cancellations are days missed from work for parents, or days away from other children at home. It's not fair, and all we can do sometimes is shrug our shoulders and say, 'That's the way it is – sorry.'

I went with the cardiac surgical registrar to inform the unlucky parents that their five-month-old would not be having surgery today. They were disappointed, but not angry, and understood. I was glad I had given my disclaimer earlier that morning. They have been given a provisional day for surgery next week, then they'll play bed roulette all over again.

41 – There Is a Fracture, I Need to Fix It

Today was another landmark in the life of a new consultant, my first weekend day 'on call'. On a normal weekday, most emergencies are completed by 6 p.m., with perhaps one or two pending. At the weekend, though, each morning you walk into whatever awaits, with no help. It is me against the world. One anaesthetist to rule them all. Only one operating theatre to do it in. Surgeons from all areas of the hospital appear from cracks in the wall. They all want in to the emergency theatre. They all have emergency cases to do. Even the radiologists might chance their arm for general anaesthesia to facilitate a scan. Orthopaedic surgeons have bones to fix, general surgeons have bowels to inspect, ENT surgeons have Lego to remove from ears, noses or throats, plastic surgeons have fingertips to reattach, gastroenterologists might be armed with cameras to insert into dark orifices, cardiac surgeons might have life-saving surgery to perform.

My job as the consultant anaesthetist is to essentially prioritise, delegate, negotiate, plead and coordinate all the cases for theatre. This requires gathering as much information as possible about the children, determining who is the 'sickest', determining who is ready to go, considering what surgery needs to be performed in a specific theatre, maximising the nursing resources that are available and coordinating post-operative plans to ensure the patient has a suitable bed and ward to go to. I must admit, it is helpful that most paediatric surgeons are very understanding and are happy to go with the order the anaesthetist thinks is most appropriate.

However, in other hospitals, I have been shouted at, put under pressure and even straight up lied to about the status of a patient by surgeons. In an unnamed hospital, an unnamed surgeon announced that there was a seven-year-old with a broken arm who needed surgery urgently, the reason being that there was 'neuro-vascular compromise' – this means the nerves and blood supply to the arm were potentially damaged due to the fracture and thus it needed to be fixed quickly to avoid further complications. There are some time-sensitive buzzwords that surgeons know will put a fire under an anaesthetist's backside and ensure they agree to anaesthe-tise a patient quickly: 'neurovascular compromise' is the buzzword for orthopaedic surgery; 'possible torsion' are the magic words for a urologist; 'category 1 Caesarean section' in obstetrics; 'ischaemic limb' in vascular surgery. Finally, 'we are doing CPR' gets me moving fairly quickly for cardiac surgery.

'There looks to be neurovascular compromise,' my orthopaedic colleague stated assertively.

'OK, no problem. What ward is she in?'

'The ED, but we can go straight to theatre from there, as it is urgent.'

'OK, we'll send for her now.'

Ring ring.

'Hello, ED, can you send Molly to theatre please?'

'Who?'

'You know, seven-year-old Molly? She's in a bad way with her broken arm.'

'There's no seven-year-old here with a broken arm.'

'You must be mistaken. The surgeon said she's been admitted, we've seen her x-ray.'

'Nope! 'fraid not, my friend.'

As it turns out, this hospital in question takes orthopaedic referrals from many other hospitals in the region. Our pal had merely been scrolling through all the x-rays for this vast catchment area (they're conveniently all on one radiology system), spotted a broken arm, saw the time and thought it would be nice to get this done before he clocked out and therefore not have to deal with it tomorrow. The child was in the ED of a hospital 90 km away. No orthopaedic surgeon had even laid eyes on the child yet, let alone diagnosed the 'neurovascular compromise' that would make this a true emergency. I did my best to give him a stern talking-to about abusing the system, but his cheeky grin told me this wasn't the first time and probably wouldn't be the last time he would try and pull a fast one.

Our day took a natural enough path and the cases seemed to prioritise themselves. We started with minor trauma (usually plastic surgery and orthopaedics) before the general surgeons completed their ward rounds. General surgeons, on call, are mostly dealing with abdominal problems. Their field is dynamic in that a child's condition is often monitored closely, in real time, before deciding if surgery is appropriate. In contrast, an orthopaedic surgeon knows immediately if an operation is required or not. If the decision is made by general surgeons to proceed, then they need surgery sooner rather than later. We followed on from trauma with several sick general surgery patients for laparotomies (open abdominal surgery).

While it is nice to be asked about how I would like to prioritise the cases, it can be difficult choosing one over the other, especially if you have not been following a patient's course in hospital closely, like the surgeons have been doing. Difficult decisions are sometimes required and having two true emergencies appear concurrently is something every anaesthetist hopes to avoid at all costs. We finished in theatre at 10 p.m. and were not called back after midnight. One more hurdle complete.

45 – Exorcism

Anaesthesia literally means: without ('an') feeling ('-aesthesia'). Therefore, a successful anaesthetic is one where the patient is unconscious, has no memory of the procedure (amnesia) and has adequate pain relief (analgesia). Unconsciousness and amnesia are a certainty if the anaesthetic has been delivered correctly. Analgesia can be a bit harder to get right as everyone perceives pain differently. But more often than not, we provide excellent pain relief.

Anaesthesia is also responsible for a number of other perioperative outcomes beyond pain relief. We also take ownership of post-operative nausea and vomiting. Any unforeseen airway complications are usually fair game for an anaesthesia audit. But even within anaesthesia, different subspecialties monitor different post-operative outcomes. Things we like to keep an eye on in paediatric anaesthesia specifically include our day-case surgery rate (where the child doesn't have to stay overnight); pre-operative fasting times; desaturation events in recovery, as kids are more prone to airway complications post-op; how fast kids return to normal behaviour; and the incidence of emergence delirium (when they 'emerge' from a state of anaesthesia).

Delirium is an acute-onset disturbed state of mind characterised by restlessness, confusion, agitation and incoherence. We often see it in patients suffering from severe infection or drug intoxication, particularly in elderly patients. In fact, elderly patients can become delirious simply by being in an environment that is unfamiliar to them. Everyone probably knows a relative who has experienced delirium in the hospital setting. Children can suffer from emergence delirium: they may be inconsolable, appear confused or irritated and their behaviour may be different from normal, like displaying aggressive tendencies.

'What's the big deal?' I hear you ask. 'You'll see the same behaviour outside every nightclub from Derry to Cork on a Saturday night.' Yes, you do indeed, but that is as a result of alcohol intoxication. Alcohol is a depressant drug, with the ability to affect behaviour and cognition, much like our anaesthetic drugs. Our delirious kids look like drunk kids. It is dangerous for the child to be in a state of delirium, as they may hurt themselves by pulling off monitoring, IV cannulas or disrupting the surgical site. Moreover, it is extremely distressing for parents to see their kid in a completely unrecognisable state. And the kids can go fucking ballistic to be fair.

Today I had to deal with possibly the worst emergence delirium I have ever seen. Liam was in hospital to have his tonsils out. He awoke from anaesthesia quietly, only to rapidly descend into deep delirium. He had a recent history of this, following another general anaesthetic, so I expected it to recur. It can be hard to manage, treat or prevent in someone who is susceptible, but there are some measures that can make it less likely. I altered my drug cocktail accordingly, but my plan bombed impressively. His wide-eyed daze seemed to peer straight through myself and his mother. He looked downright demonic as he repeated the same phrase over and over and over again. He screamed at his mother and punched and slapped his father repeatedly, just for being nearby. Then he pulled his mother close, only to shove her away moments later. After 45 minutes of trying various other drugs and failing, I felt powerless. His parents looked at me for a solution that I honestly didn't have. A quick fix would be to re-anaesthetise him, but this would be merely kicking the can down the road. Then, a break in the clouds. His speech became more coherent, the punching ceased and he asked for food. Mum produced a doughnut the size of his head. He went to work on it – and that was it. Not a peep more out of him. For me, this was a failed anaesthetic, a poor outcome. I felt terrible for the parents. I apologised for them having to see him like this. His mother replied, 'That was way better than the last time! He could've got a role in *The Omen* after the last anaesthetic.'

50 – Bacterial Bonanza

Yes, yes, yes – I understand that we will all die of a bacterial apocalypse in the future, but why is preventing such an event so *annoying*? A threat that you cannot see, smell, hear, touch or taste is hard to fathom as a threat at all. Climate change is the quintessential example of this. It's happening, but I can't experience it progressing on a daily basis. If much of the most powerful nation on Earth doesn't even acknowledge its existence, what chance have you got of convincing Kurt from Springfield, USA that he probably doesn't really need a 6.0-litre pick-up truck?

The hospital version of climate change is bacterial resistance. It's a crisis that we all acknowledge is happening, and we all do what we can to prevent it. Our methods of doing so, however, are occasionally inconsistent, and sometimes comical. There are many 'superbugs' as the tabloids like to call them – MRSA, VRE, CRE, EBSL, ABBA … LOL … WTF … OMG. Many people are colonised by these bacteria. The key thing for people to understand is that colonisation is not the same as infection. If you are colonised, the bacteria sit harmlessly on your skin or in your nose, reading the newspaper and minding their own business.

If a person becomes unwell, and their immune system becomes compromised, or they have an invasive surgical procedure, then these bacteria may become a problem and can potentially cause an infection. An infection results in fever, pus and generalised sickness. A proven bacterial infection is treated with antibiotics. The problem with the 'superbugs' is that standard antibiotics don't work on them any more, as these particular bugs have evolved over time to become resistant. Their evolution is far quicker than any other species because there are just so many of the little monsters and they reproduce rapidly, so they can change rapidly. For some infectious bacteria, we are down to our very last effective antibiotics. For some of the superbugs, we have no antibiotics left. There could be a point in the future where people could die from a cut on their finger, tonsillitis or the good, old-fashioned clap.

The thing is that each individual hospital is like its own bacterial ecosystem. Where one hospital has MRSA, another has none. Where one has CRE, another doesn't. Every hospital has an infection-control team that are tasked with protecting the hospital from bugs from other hospitals and also protecting the patients from each other. This involves all your standard things – washing hands, wearing gowns and gloves, isolating patients who are known to be colonised with a particular bacteria. While it is absolutely necessary, it is a hugely time-consuming process to manage in an operating theatre.

If a patient comes for surgery who is known to be colonised, all unnecessary equipment is removed from the theatre, everyone dons gowns and gloves, the patient must not go into an area where there are other patients and the operating theatre is closed after that particular case in order to undergo a very thorough clean. All understandable. But, we have got to the point now where patients who have potentially, maybe, sort of, kinda been in contact with someone who is colonised also have to be treated as infectious in theatre. For example, our hospital has no CRE (carbapenem-resistant enterobacteriaceae, if you're so inclined). If you have *ever* attended a hospital where there had been CRE, you are treated as a 'CRE precaution' and thus all the rigmarole in theatre kicks in. If you drove to the car park of a CRE hospital – CRE precautions. If you had a dream about maybe going to a CRE hospital – CRE precautions. If you learned the word for hospital in Portuguese – CRE precautions. If your great-grandfather was stationed in the South Pacific in the Second World War – CRE precautions.

Of our seven cases today, three were treated as CRE precautions. That meant a 30-minute operation became a 90-minute operation, as the child must recover in the operating room, instead of the recovery area, in order to reduce the chances of another child becoming colonised, even if the patient isn't known to be colonised by CRE. The operating theatre is then thoroughly cleaned (don't worry, we always clean it, just *really* well after an infectious case) each time. It can sometimes grind theatre activity to a halt, and it will only get worse over time as more and more bacteria fall into the unfortunately named 'superbug' category. It is very much a crisis, and is not sustainable in the long term. From the operating theatre perspective, we will simply run out of time, on any given day, to perform all the scheduled surgeries if every patient was colonised by some unwanted bacteria.

The infection-control team has a tough job, to be fair, but the management can be confusing. I recall starting work in another hospital and infection control decided to swab all the new doctors. Ordinarily, if someone is positive for MRSA, they are isolated (or removed from the hospital) and undergo a decontamination regimen before being swabbed again to remove the MRSA positive status. So many of the new doctors had positive nasal swabs for MRSA, myself included, that the hospital would cease to function if they prevented us all from working. So we went to work. I recall treating a child with potential tuberculosis who had been isolated during her entire stay in the hospital. The day she was discharged (still with possible tuberculosis) she hopped on the rush-hour train home from Waterloo Station with her mum. On a daily basis, we clear theatres out of all but necessary equipment for an 'infected' case, but whatever items cannot be moved out get draped with large sheets of almost transparent porous tissue paper. God help us if our last line of defence is flimsy tissue paper that rather sizeable ants could casually saunter through.

There is some lesson I'm trying to convey with this microbiological anecdote, but I'm not sure what it is. 'Enjoy your last days on Earth as soon you'll be dead from the common cold!' Too grim. 'Please ensure that you perform rectal swabs on you and your family members when leaving the hospital.' Unlikely to catch on. 'Don't go to Spain as you'll catch the flesh-eating bacteria!' No. Ok, ok, ok – please take your antibiotics as directed by your doctor, don't ask for antibiotics for mild illnesses that are most likely viral, wash your hands in the hospital (well, always wash your hands) and make sure you tell the hospital if you know you are colonised with a specific bacteria.

51 – Chicken Fillet Baguettes

Ear, nose and throat (ENT) surgeons operate on the ear, nose and throat – congratulations, you're ready to be a doctor! I've always thought their name was interesting. You don't call the orthopaedic surgeon the 'arm, leg and spine' surgeon. Or the urologist the 'kidney, bladder and prostate' surgeon (and realistically, if we were re-naming urologists, one would naturally focus on the genitalia – 'Hi, I'm Dr Dick Steel, cock doctor'). But the official name for ENT surgery is otolaryngology which is a bit of a mouthful and I've just realised it completely omits the poor nose from the equation: it's otorhinolaryngology if you feel the nose is deserving a mention. ENT surgery ranges from some of the most straightforward cases you could think of (e.g. placing an ear grommet, which takes approximately 60 seconds) to some of the most complex. In adults, complex procedures include operations to remove a patient's entire larynx (voice box) for a cancer that is affecting their ability to breathe. In kids, complex cases can involve diagnosing or treating some congenital problem that affects the child's ability to breathe effectively. It makes for truly frightening anaesthesia, but it is amazing work and these surgeons have large *cojones*. Today, though, we are mostly performing E surgery – just the ear.

My registrar is having lunch, so I anaesthetise a little girl for an ear operation on my own. She is a low-risk, healthy child, and mere seconds after I have anaesthetised her, her parents leave through one door and my registrar returns through another, like a well-choreographed theatre transition (the other kind of theatre). I leave my registrar in peace and take the chance to head off to grab a sandwich. Naturally, as soon as I walk into the hospital café I walk straight into the parents of said child, who is still under anaesthesia upstairs. *Oh Jesus, I told them I'd be there the whole time! Or did I tell them myself or my registrar would be there the whole time?* Of course, they never actually met my registrar so as far as they're concerned, the man tasked with preserving the life of their dearest has abandoned his post in search of a chicken fillet baguette. Here I am, licking my lips at the sight of that warm, tender chicken, unsure of what to do. Do I explain myself? Do I apologise? Can I expect a complaint? Do I buy them a sandwich? We all look at each other awkwardly. A short silence.

'All is going well up there!' I open with, forgetting the fact that I literally walked down here as fast as they could have, and there is no way the ENT surgeon has even put on a pair of gloves yet.

'Thanks for everything, doctor. Looks like a busy day. Enjoy your lunch!'

I realise I've probably reinforced the myth that anaesthetists merely inject people and leave the room for coffee instantaneously.

52 – Mistaken Identity

'You're the surgical SHO aren't you?'
'How many more years of anaesthesia training do you have?'
'How did you get on in Canada? When did you get back?'
'What consultant are you with today?'
'Can you please start admitting the surgery day cases?'
Now I don't know how many men, around 6 foot tall, with a short beard there are in the world, but apparently there are bloody loads of them in this hospital. The phrases above represent the cases of mistaken identity I have endured in the last two weeks alone. According to many nurses, I am not who I think I am. I am the general surgery SHO, an anaesthetic registrar, a former colleague who worked in Canada, another anaesthetic registrar and the general surgery SHO again. They really wish me to be the general surgery SHO. You could forgive someone for doing it once, but multiple times seems a bit unnecessary, considering I do wear an identification badge around my neck in plain sight.

I don't really mind the mistaken identity; I am only two months into the job and the permanent hospital staff has to deal with all the new medical faces every few months as trainees rotate through the hospital. But on the flipside, I have worked here before – a couple of times. I do get a little kick out of it, though, I must say. It's particularly fun on the surgical day unit which is as busy as Heathrow Airport in the morning. The head nurses in the unit run a tight ship and tell the junior doctors exactly who needs to be admitted in the morning and who needs to be reviewed by anaesthesia. They are not quite but *verging* on bossy:

'Which consultant anaesthetist are you with today? You're going to have to get them to review this child, they are quite complex.'

'Em, I am the consultant ...'

'Ohhhh, sorry, sorry, sorry!'

'Will you get in there and do that child's consent form quickly, they'll be calling from theatre soon.'

'I'm the consultant anaesthetist ...'

'OH. MY. GOD. I'm sorry. You really look like the surgical SHO.'

I might throw a few curveballs into the mix in the next couple of weeks.

'I'm a medical student.'

'My twin brother is the general surgery SHO.'

'You probably recognise me from *Dancing with the Stars*.'

'Oh! I'm just here looking for morphine.'

'Can you believe they managed to rescue me from that mine?'

58 – A Different Kind of DNA

Our single MRI machine is hot property. If it were on Tinder, it would be matching with prospective partners all day long. *Patient Larry sent you a message: 'Are you free this afternoon?'* If we could sell tickets to see the MRI machine, the prices would be at World

Cup final level. *Patient Kate has offered €2,500 for a 60-minute slot.* If the MRI machine were walking down Oxford Street, the paparazzi would be falling over each other. Patient Amy screams, *'MRI! MRI! Over here, look at me!'* An audience with the MRI machine would have more attendees than the Pope's visit to Dublin in 1979. Patient Jason solemnly proclaims, *'Your MRI Holiness, I have been waiting for this day for years.'* Time in our MRI machine is so scarce that no one in their right mind would fail to show up for an appointment. Except they do, every day.

The MRI list is always busy. Every single minute is accounted for so we can cram as much scanning as is humanly possible into the day. The plan today is two walk-in scans (as in no general anaesthesia required) followed by five scans under general anaesthesia, one more walk-in over lunch, three more under general anaesthesia in the afternoon and another walk-in to finish. Twelve or so MRI scans in total. We pray there are no emergency scans requested from the wards or intensive care, as MRI scans are not quick – they last anywhere from 15 to 90 minutes for complex imaging.

Last week, the MRI machine broke down and caused chaos for about 24 hours. Imagine buying a ten-year-old car and driving it, continuously, from Dublin to Cork for ten hours a day, every day, without stopping for a service until you hit the 300,000-kilometre mark. It will break down, that much is guaranteed. When the car is repaired, suddenly there are 25 hitchhikers all demanding the first lift back to Dublin.

Many of the kids who need general anaesthesia for an MRI scan are not particularly well. They can be hazardous to anaesthetise in an area that is away from the main theatre block. It would be easy to lose focus and make a clinical or judgement error when the service demands rapid anaesthesia. We are motoring (relating back to my car analogy – thanks) through the first few general anaesthetics (GAs) but then have an unexpected airway complication anaesthetising the third child. This sets us back on our schedule by 15 minutes. *It feels warm in here.* I want to get all these kids scanned today. The last GA before lunch is a complicated child with hypertrophic obstructive cardiomyopathy (HOCM).[23] HOCM is probably one of the most worrying and difficult cardiac diagnoses to safely anaesthetise. A severe HOCM could easily suffer a cardiac arrest under anaesthesia. I have spent most of the morning mulling over my plan for this one. A lot of preparation is needed but we successfully anaesthetise the child with still one eye on the clock. But it's not ideal doing that one on the clock.

The afternoon rolls around and our next patient is not in the hospital. Not only that, but the one after also didn't show up. The consultant radiologist is in the MRI control room waiting. The radiographers are all ready to work. We are waiting to anaesthetise these kids. The waiting time for an outpatient MRI scan under general anaesthesia is several *years* (at the time of writing). Years. We contact the day unit and ask if they've heard from the children's parents. Nothing. Not a peep. All parents are called and reminded of the appointment date and time in the days before the scheduled MRI. Both of these parents received a call the day before and they confirmed they would be attending on time.

As we see in the news every day, waiting times for all hospital services are scandalously long. Today's figure in the newspaper stated that there were 500,000 people waiting for outpatient clinic appointments. Certainly, we don't have enough staff, time or

---

23 Hypertrophic obstructive cardiomyopathy (HOCM) is a rare congenital cardiac disease. Medical terms are usually fairly self-explanatory when you know the basics of their Latin origins. A cardiomyopathy is literally 'disease of the heart muscle'. Hypertrophic means 'thickening' and obstructive means obstructive. In HOCM, parts of the left ventricle can become so hypertrophied that the opposing walls of the ventricle can come into contact as the heart beats causing obstruction to blood flow. It puts a lot of strain on the heart muscle to generate force to expel the blood effectively. It leaves sufferers at high risk of sudden cardiac death.

resources currently to significantly reduce these outrageous waiting times. However, there should be some accountability on patients too. All outpatient clinics have multiple 'DNA' stamps in the clinical notes. DNA = did not attend. A DNA without a call or a letter or any attempt to get in contact with the hospital. A DNA without any thought for the doctors, nurses and secretaries expecting them or who have to chase them afterwards to rearrange an appointment. Most tellingly, a DNA without any thought for the fact that another person, waiting patiently, could have had their slot in clinic or had their MRI scan.

This is not the first time that a lack of punctuality or even some common decency has got me seething. I don't think I'm a bad person for this annoying me. I think of the kid who has been patiently waiting for a scan. I think of the nurses who have been working with me at a rate of knots this morning without a break to keep things moving. And selfishly, I think of myself. Knowing we had a cancellation could have given me more time to prepare for a tricky anaesthetic. Our system may be breaking, but there is onus on the patients to do their part too.

59 – The Conservative Party

For the registrars I imagine I am still a bit of a nightmare to work with. At this stage, I'm still not used to having a junior colleague in theatre with me. I'm used to working solo and, frankly, I sometimes have the urge to work solo. I'm not saying the registrars are incapable of doing things; quite the opposite actually – many of them are excellent. The thing that I'm struggling a bit with is allowing them some independence. I've come to realise the main difference in being a registrar and consultant is the burden of responsibility. Now, all the responsibility lies with me. As a good registrar you are capable of performing well in almost all aspects of the job, but you can always ask the consultant for help. I have found myself, so far, choosing to perform most of the higher-risk procedural elements to the job (e.g. intubating the small babies, performing regional anaesthesia) myself. This is because I know I can do it and I want it to be successful the first time. I am risk averse at the best of times (a trait that is probably desirable in your anaesthetist), but even more so in the early months in the hot seat. My ubiquitous presence must be infuriating for the more senior registrars who are itching to get this kind of experience without me meddling in their opportunities.

It is this desire for good outcomes that makes me slightly more conservative now compared to just a few months ago in my life as a senior registrar or fellow. I was always baffled when I saw a junior consultant digging deep into a patient history before a minor procedure or getting lots of fancy equipment out to help with what I perceived to be a simple airway to manage. But now I understand. I don't want to miss an iota in the patient notes and I particularly don't want to experience any major complications. A few cases have already tested my skills in the last couple of months and I now err more on the conservative side than before. I'm sure that once I get my footing this will change for the better.

The more senior consultant anaesthetists are more relaxed and allow the registrars more independence – 'You want to make the trainees sweat, just a little bit' was one take on it. I will certainly get to that stage, but only when I feel ready. It's reassuring to hear a senior colleague admit to me that the 'scary' cases don't ever go away, they just become less frequent.

64 – Language Matters

'We have an issue with consent.'

This is a common phrase, heard most days in the operating theatre, usually prompting the anaesthetist to roll their eyes to heaven, wondering how it's possible that the surgical team have failed to obtain consent for surgery from their patients. Without a signed consent form, we cannot bring any child to the operating theatre, unless it is a life-threatening emergency. This lack of a signed consent form is usually a result of the surgical team being tied up and scrubbed in the operating theatre; i.e. they can't go haring around the hospital with a clipboard looking for the parents. In their defence, they gain consent from as many patients as possible in the morning. Being scrubbed precludes them from seeing any late-arriving patients until they are free. Our issue with consent today was a little different. The child's family weren't native English speakers, and although they spoke some English it was questionable whether it was sufficient to understand a complex medical procedure. Their child had a history of congenital scoliosis and was due to have growth rods inserted into the spine. This is not a typical level of vocabulary in a new language, and hardly something they're chatting about with the neighbours in Tesco. Even describing the procedure to a native English speaker can be difficult, and requires a significant degree of understanding.

Consent in medicine should be 'informed consent'. This is the process of laying it all out on the table for the patient and their families: explaining the diagnosis, discussing all the available treatment options and discussing the likely progression of the condition should they not proceed with treatment. Once a treatment is selected and agreed upon, all possible risks and side effects are discussed. Ideally, the patient and family are given ample time to ask questions and mull it over before signing a consent form. In some cases it's a no-brainer – you have appendicitis, so you agree to have an appendicectomy, otherwise you might get very septic and die. The benefit of removing the infected appendix outweighs the risk of leaving it in, or any risk of a surgical complication. Most situations aren't quite as straightforward, but it is always a similar decision-making process: a balancing act that you hope will weigh down on the side of benefit over risk.

The consent process is not always ideal in medicine; one could argue that requesting consent only 30 minutes before an operation doesn't give the patient ample time to really consider the risks. While patients have the right to determine their treatment course, many defer to the opinion of the medical expert. This is absolutely fine, provided they have been given all the necessary information and, crucially, they understand it. The doctor and patient must agree on what outcomes are expected. Fully informed consent therefore, especially for major surgery, should not be easy listening, and the decision to proceed should not be taken lightly.

Surgery requires anaesthesia, therefore the consent to undergo anaesthesia is usually implied by the decision to sign a consent form for surgery; there is no specific consent form. Regardless of this, anaesthetists will always explain to the patient what they will be doing, and what to expect. I try to be very thorough, and this occasionally results in parents crying. A senior colleague of mine in London once told me that if the parents weren't crying after signing consent for any paediatric heart operation, then they haven't fully understood the procedure and therefore it isn't fully informed consent. Naturally, the goal wasn't to make people cry, but the gravity and seriousness of the operation should be laid out plain and simple.

I will often see that a proactive surgical team member has included the 'risk of anaesthesia' in their consent for surgery. I am always happy to see this, as it shows that they appreciate that there is no surgery without anaesthesia. Its inclusion also plays to our inferiority complex and makes us feel slightly more important. 'Risk of anaesthesia' is often followed by the statistic '1/10,000'. I have seen this written so many times that I am certain that surgeons are taught it. The risk of anaesthesia is 1/10,000? What does that even mean? 1/10,000 die? Not true. 1/10,000 have a failed anaesthetic? Not true. 1/10,000 cannot spell anaesthesia? Not true, that's way more common. 1/10,000 will experience Nirvana? Don't think so. The fact is that anaesthesia is *extremely* safe for the standard patient. Dying from anaesthesia *alone* is so very rare that it is likely I will never see this in my career. We're talking close to a one-in-a-million territory. Yes it is true that anaesthesia alone brings risks of relatively minor things like nausea or vomiting (probably 1/10) or risks of more serious things like malignant hyperthermia (1/100,000) – but death? Not so.[24]

If more serious complications occur after surgery, they are usually as a result of the patient's pre-operative condition or how the surgery has affected the physiology of the body. In the elective setting, it is mostly your cardio-respiratory fitness that determines your risk. Surgery, by its very nature, is an assault on the body. It activates your fight-or-flight response. If you struggle to climb the stairs without getting short of breath, how will your body cope with a major surgical assault? Major emergency surgery results in more post-operative complications and carries with it a higher morbidity and mortality. This is usually because the patient is suffering from something very acutely wrong with them (a perforated bowel, a major trauma), putting them in a higher risk category as they are starting from a significantly worse position of health than those who are having planned surgery. Combine poor cardio-respiratory health with major emergency surgery and you could be looking at a long stay in intensive care. It is the recovery from surgery that is the hardest part of the peri-operative journey. Yes, in the operating theatre setting our anaesthetic drugs can make a sick person sicker, but we always consider these risks and mitigate

---

24 Malignant hyperthermia (MH) is a rare, abnormal reaction to some anaesthetic drugs as a result of a genetic abnormality in a specific receptor in your muscle cells. It is serious and can be life threatening but can be managed effectively, making death extremely rare. If we know someone carries the abnormal gene, then we can alter our technique and make anaesthesia perfectly safe. It can run in families, so we test siblings and offspring when a case of MH presents itself.

as best we can to facilitate surgery. Often we can predict, accurately, who will be unstable and sick after their surgery. This is why we have intensive care units.[25]

The standard for consenting a patient who speaks little or no English would be to use a certified interpreter. However, today none were available. On hearing this, our surgeon, as well as a nurse on the ward, attempted to use their Leaving Cert language skills to explain a complicated orthopaedic operation. There were drawings everywhere. Crayons on the floor. Google Translate was in overdrive. It can't have been reassuring for the poor mother. Alas, after the effort, it was felt that there was not enough comprehension and so the procedure was cancelled for today. We will reschedule for when an interpreter is available.

71 – Gender Identity

The functions of the theatre porter are as follows: motivator, psychologist, mindfulness coach and transporter. In that order. And that's just for the other staff, never mind the kids. Each child's first encounter with a strange person in blue pyjamas is usually with the theatre porter who arrives on the ward to collect them for surgery. In addition, they are always the last person in blue pyjamas that a child sees after surgery, signalling the end of their theatre experience. They bookend the day in theatre for the kids. Naturally, inquisitive children pepper the porters with questions before and after surgery. They seem to be comfortable and chatty with the

---

25 I have been discussing in this paragraph how the patient's health affects risk. There are, of course, additional risks of technical surgical complications that I have not addressed, but these are thoroughly explained by surgeons in the consent process. To go further, although a broken finger or a cut on your foot may require 'emergency' surgery, these minor things don't affect your overall health, therefore add no additional risk. Not all 'emergency' surgery is in the same risk bracket.

porters' questions but can immediately become shy and coy when a person identifying themselves as the doctor arrives. When I was a kid, a mention of 'the doctor' was almost threatening or sinister. 'Behave yourself for the doctor!' Or occasionally, 'OK, if you're really sick I'm taking you to the doctor!', to which the reply was always, 'No, I'm fine!'

Calming children in unfamiliar environments is a talent, and some of our porters are experts. They have seen enough surgery to explain exactly what will happen without the doctors butting in. They have sometimes done half my job for me. Preparing a child for theatre starts long before the journey to theatre begins and the porters (and anaesthetic nurses) handle the last preparatory hurdle before a child embarks on their journey into the unknown. Naturally, we don't always welcome a perfectly chilled-out kid to theatre; the occasion can get the better of them. It's then down to us, as anaesthetists, to make the last effort to put them at ease and make the task of inducing anaesthesia as smooth as possible. As a registrar, I regularly observed a senior anaesthetist calming down even the most raucous and resistant children into compliant and beaming angels. His approach is multi-faceted; it's in his tone of voice, his stance and his gaze, a wonderful talent honed over many years, and something I strive to match.

On leaving theatre, groggy children enjoy bizarre conversations with porters that they will never remember. But the porters play along with the stories, or kids' interpretation of what they just experienced. Our overwhelmingly male porters relentlessly joke with the kids and, more frequently, take the piss out of each other. They don't let each other get away with anything. You can hear their voices booming at each other around the entire theatre complex. The partner of one of our porters is expecting a baby. Unfortunately for him, on several occasions today we all heard him getting excited about going on his maternity leave. He left himself wide open to be taken to the cleaners by his quick-witted portering pals.

'Jesus Christ, not again. *PAT*ernity leave, you get *PAT*ernity leave. Think of your Uncle Pat, is he a man? Yes. Pat gets paternity leave.'

73 – Collaborative Multi-Faceted Task Dispersal and Resolution

Being an anaesthetist is very much being part of a team, a cohesive group with a common goal. Our focus every day is to facilitate as much surgery as possible and, in doing so, minimise how much theatre activity occurs outside normal working hours. It is far safer to work in daylight hours with well-slept, alert and enthusiastic staff, with back-up in the adjacent room, than red-eyed, hungry and error-prone staff after midnight.

As I started my elective (scheduled) cardiac surgery cases today, I made the foolish move of peering at the emergency board. Eleven cases plastered across it already, and it was only 8 a.m. Even with a dedicated emergency theatre working full steam ahead, it would be tricky to complete them by day's end. I had a vested interest in the swell of the emergency list, as I'm on call tonight. Any emergency cases not completed in normal working hours would be left to me to perform after a long day of work. Trying to sneak a couple of emergencies into a vacant theatre also looks improbable as we are working with a full complement of open theatres today, all with their own sizeable elective lists to work through.

The long emergency list is compounded by the fact that I know I will have to anaesthetise an infant for an emergency cardiac procedure tonight. The family is not yet in the hospital but the case is already tickling the worry lobe of my brain. Ideally, this would be the only case I would have to deal with tonight. I try to put the pile of emergencies out of my head, focus on the child in front of me and hope my colleagues deal with them during the course of the day.

We use the term 'emergency' just to differentiate from 'elective'. In truth, not all emergencies are 'true' emergencies in the sense that they have to be rushed, *ER* style, off the ambulance or chopper, through the corridors and straight into theatre. True emergencies do occur, but most 'emergencies' would be better described as 'urgent' – they ideally need to be done within 12 to 24 hours or so. You can tell what time of year it is by the emergency list. Broken wrists and busted lips are summer injuries as the trampolines get pulled out in back gardens when the good weather appears. We can defer some 'emergencies' to the following day, but the aim is always to get as much done as possible on the same day. No one is going to die from a broken arm while in hospital, but a child is in pain and needs an operation.

If elective lists finish early, there is scope to do emergency cases in that theatre if the appropriate surgeon is available and the anaesthetist agrees. I think of what a manager might call this. *Dynamic theatre utility. Maximisation of blue-sky opportunity. Collaborative multi-faceted task dispersal and resolution.*

At 2 p.m. it still looks shit. The assigned emergency theatre is occupied for the rest of the day with a major case. But by 4 p.m., miraculously, it's looking good. There are now four emergency cases on the list. My colleagues and team-mates are pressing on, utilising multi-angles to collaboratively dynamite the resolute night sky.

By 6 p.m., I'm finished and, by some miracle, almost all the emergency cases are done. It is just the little baby I was expecting remaining. My long night suddenly seems more manageable, and we can take our time and fully concentrate on our last tiny patient without any distractions. This is only possible due to the collective effort of my colleagues who took on an extra case or two in order to minimise the work of the on-call consultant. I look at tomorrow's emergency list; it has now swollen (pun intended) to 11 fractures. It looks like we'll be calling the same team effort into action again tomorrow.

78 – CP

Cerebral palsy is a common condition to encounter in a children's hospital, but I think it is probably one of the most misunderstood medical conditions by the general public. The crux of this misunderstanding is the fact that the severity of cerebral palsy (or CP for short) is very much on a scale. It is a condition linked to a brain injury occurring late in pregnancy, during a difficult labour or in the first precarious few weeks of life. This resultant deficit is caused primarily by a period of lack of oxygen to the brain or sometimes by severe infection.[26] The phrase 'cerebral palsy' really doesn't tell you anything about how it affects someone. 'Cerebral' refers to the largest part of the brain known as the cerebrum. It looks firm but, according to the neurosurgeons, it's really quite gelatinous. The cerebrum is the outer part of brain tissue that appears like folded waves of soft cheese and it controls many motor and sensory functions. The 'palsy', while usually meaning paralysis, in this context essentially means 'problem'. Therefore, CP manifests differently from person to person, depending on what specific area of the brain has been affected and how extensive the damage. It commonly causes physical problems that can affect mobility and speech but can also affect cognitive processing too. There are patterns of CP symptoms that can be similar from person to person (e.g. spasticity – the rigid muscle contractions that can result in fixed, abnormal and uncomfortable postures), but this doesn't necessarily match their level of disability. It is very difficult to foresee how an early diagnosis of CP will affect a child's ability to function in the future, as their symptoms can evolve or improve over time, due to the plasticity of a child's brain.

You can meet someone who has very subtle CP that you'd have to observe very closely to spot any sign of a problem. Conversely,

---

26 There are other, rare causes also.

you can meet someone who is very profoundly disabled and unable to perform any physical tasks or communicate effectively. I don't want to make light of CP as it is a life-changing diagnosis, but often the general public assumes that a diagnosis of CP means there is no hope for a child to attend school or become independent. This is not the case.

We had two fantastic kids with CP for MRI scans today. The differences between them demonstrate, firstly, the spectrum of the disease and, secondly, how physical appearances can be deceiving. One should not jump to conclusions about someone with a disability. Our first child was Alex, who was wheelchair-bound, nonverbal (unable to speak) and in need of full-time care at home. He had suffered from seizures for a lot of his life, but these were now increasing in frequency and severity, justifying an MRI of his brain. He had been anaesthetised many times before for various orthopaedic procedures to relieve the inevitable muscular contractures that develop when wheelchair-bound with CP and the associated spasticity. I introduce myself to his parents and himself. He reaches for my ID badge and starts beaming from ear to ear. I use a stethoscope to listen to his chest and he turns to his parents appearing thrilled with the visit from the doctor. He never takes his eyes off me. If only all the kids were as happy to see me.

Our second child is Harry, who has a diagnosis of ataxic CP. Ataxia causes a person to have uncoordinated movement of muscle, commonly while walking or speaking. It can indicate damage to the cerebellum, another part of the brain that looks a bit like a cauliflower, which controls coordinated movement.[27] On first glance he is sitting playing dextrously with some Lego blocks while making all the appropriate chatter one would expect of his age. When he sees me approaching he pops up off the floor and hurries over to

---

27 Alcohol affects the cerebellum, which is why you often see drunk people staggering or walking strangely.

the safety of Mum, and it's only then that I note a very subtle abnormality in his gait (his walking pattern) that suggests something is not quite right. It isn't obvious, though; even a medical student might miss it.

Certainly before I studied medicine and rotated to a paediatric hospital as a student, I assumed that CP meant full-time care and a low quality of life – how naïve I was. The concept of 'quality of life' is one that comes up across all medical specialties, as any chronic illnesses can impede one's quality of life, and treatment aims to improve this. Adults and those kids who can communicate well can reliably inform you of their quality of life: which things have improved, and which are still a struggle. It is easy to assume that those who are very young or those who can't communicate verbally (such as Alex, above) have a poor quality of life, but when you meet kids like Alex, whose smile lights up the room, or Harry, whose diagnosis of CP is of no major consequence to him, then you have to think again. CP is not curable, but treatment can rehabilitate and improve functional aspects of a CP patient's life. I have great admiration for the rehabilitation medical, nursing and allied health staff (like physiotherapists and occupational therapists) who work with these kids every day, where the small changes they work on can make a huge difference in functional rehabilitation.

79 – It's Like Pulling Off a Band-Aid

Becoming a consultant means that, for the first time, I am an 'El Chapo', 'El Jefe', 'the boss' – or something like that. When you are training, you feel like part of a large trainee army (anaesthetic departments are huge), flanked by comrades senior and junior to you.[28] We provide each other with advice, help with problems and,

---

28 Anaesthesia is the largest hospital-based medical specialty. You just don't see us or remember us. *Wipes away tear.*

inevitably, bitch about the consultants. During my training I've worked with many super (and some not-so-super) consultants whose personalities varied considerably. Some were very laid back, some were hugely supportive and encouraging, some prepped me for exams, but there were others who micro-managed, others who gave out to me relentlessly and some who walked the tightrope of verbal abuse. I always wondered what these consultants were like as trainees. Were they always so picky about 'X'? Or did they give out to nursing staff about 'Y'? Or were they so chilled that they had to be dragged around by nurses to actually get some work done?

I have always tried to not get my knickers in a twist about things that were beyond my control, as so many facets of life in a hospital fall into this area. Getting frustrated about things you can't influence either way is a sure-fire way of becoming agitated and stressed. However, now that I'm a 'boss', I can influence some things a little bit more than before. I get to spend time with every trainee on a one-on-one basis and therefore can hopefully make an impact on how they approach working with me. This exposes all trainees to inevitable comparisons with their peers – in my own head only, of course. As a trainee, you don't really get a good grasp on your trainee colleagues' working attitudes or performances on the job as you very rarely spend time in the same operating theatre together. The point is not to compare people directly (who would win in a fight?) but to get a grasp on who could handle the most responsibility. My own attitude as a trainee was always to be extremely well prepared, to know everything about each patient and to have a plan in mind for how the day will run.

In my short time as a consultant, I have observed two things in the realm of trainees:

There are huge inter-trainee differences in ability. Not only in knowledge and skills, but in attitude and accountability. I'm probably more anal than I thought I was.

The reason I'm pondering this today is that I had to pull up a trainee on poor performance. I'm a very non-confrontational person, and I don't do well in arguments. Generally, I give people the benefit of the doubt, understand people can have off days and hope that a bad day was just a once-off. But as my more assertive wife pointed out, I'm not doing anyone any favours by withholding feedback if I think a trainee is being lazy, or not up to standard in any way.

No one likes giving negative feedback, and no one likes to receive it, even if it's justified. The issue today revolved around punctuality and preparedness for the working day. The registrar in question arrived 45 minutes after I did (a mere five minutes before the first patient is due in theatre), had skipped the standard morning teaching session for registrars, had no idea what operations we were performing today, despite this information being available 24 hours previously, and had not been to assess any of the patients for the list (I had met four). There was no apology or explanation.

I gritted my teeth and pondered whether I was being unreasonable. *Perhaps the traffic was bad? Maybe there are other issues going on? Maybe I'm just turning into one of those consultants I used to hate working with?* I pondered whether a private discussion with him about work expectations would subsequently be shared with other trainees and I'd be flagged as a consultant trainees don't look forward to working with. I decided that realistically the entire point of training and working with different consultants is so that trainees can grow, accept responsibility and become accountable for how they work. The endgame being becoming a consultant themselves. To that end, they should really start thinking like one. I would not be fulfilling my role as a teacher if I didn't pull trainees up on aspects of their work they need to improve upon.

I bit the bullet and calmly admitted that I was disappointed with the registrar's attitude to work. The registrar nodded in agreement and said they could do better. It was like pulling a Band-Aid off:

thinking about it was worse that actually doing it. *Have I ruined the learning environment between me and this registrar now? Will the other trainees think I'm a bit of a dick?*

My job, first and foremost, is to provide safe care to the children I am anaesthetising on a daily basis. If I thought a team member might jeopardise this high standard, I must call them out on it. It's not even a high standard; in truth, it's the minimum standard. I might reflect on some of my opinions of the fussy consultants that trained me; I think I can relate to them a bit more already.

81 – Jon Snow's Arse

Training to be a consultant, in any specialty, is a strange concept. You work for years to get a medical degree, you then work your socks off to gain a place in a post-graduate training programme and you then move yourself, and family, if applicable, around the country to work in various hospitals. You do this for six to ten years, you sit more exams, you spend long nights writing research papers, you spend your hard-earned cash to pay for trips to medical conferences you don't necessarily want to go to in order to present your work, you often are responsible for running an inpatient service on a day-to-day basis and then finally you get the precious CCST – Certificate of Completion of Specialist Training. Finally, your ticket to consultancy! Except that often there are no available consultant posts in the city you have settled your family in, that your kids to go to school in and where your partner works. In some specialties there may be no desirable posts anywhere. In others, the competition is overwhelming. What other job would someone work relentlessly for over many years only to be unemployed at the end?

It's no wonder that trainees get very strategic about their career plans. It doesn't always become a case of working in the niche you enjoy the most, but in the niche where you see the future employment opportunities. I was very fortunate in that I loved paediatric anaesthesia and there were upcoming consultant posts that timed perfectly with the end of my fellowship in London. But that is the exception, not the rule. Some specialties are slow to expand and very experienced would-be consultants literally have to wait for someone to retire ... or die. Never walk down the stairs in front of someone looking for a consultant's post.

I had a senior registrar approach me for career advice today which was simultaneously flattering and daunting. My opinion seemingly mattered greatly to this person, otherwise they would not have asked me. What I suggest could influence their career path and affect their long-term job prospects. When you reach the final year of training, everyone starts weighing up their peers, and your friends can morph into rivals for future consultant jobs. Decisions regarding fellowships abroad or further training at home need to be made. Calculations as to what subspecialty to pursue need to be balanced between desire and need. Do I suggest to someone that they pursue their vague interest in obstetric anaesthesia just because two consultants are retiring soon? Ultimately, I don't think any junior doctor does with their career precisely what any senior doctor advises. In this kind of conversation or mentoring, the best one can do is to provide someone seeking guidance with the tools to decide for themselves. Everyone's circumstances are different.

So what did I advise this person to do? Cheesily, to pursue their true passion; 'it will all work out in the end'. Suitable for the end of an episode of *Love Island*. He's now a body-double for Jon Snow in Season 8 of *Game of Thrones*, and you can see his bum in Episode 2. He's hoping his bum can take him all the way to Hollywood.

82 – Number 2

'Hi, my name is Colin and I have a problem with punctuality.'

'Welcome to your first meeting of Ageing Anaesthetists Anonymous, Colin. We'll put your problem in the OGB or "Old Grumpy Bollocks" category.'

Another day, another group of late patients. Maybe it *is* me with the problem? I know arriving late to the party on a Friday night evokes an air of mystique, like you've been somewhere painfully cool early in the evening and the hosts are lucky to bear witness to your presence at their lame party. But I'm struggling to apply this logic to hospital appointments. Now before every reader gets annoyed at me I will of course recognise the following: a) the public transport to our hospital isn't great; b) not everyone has a car; and c) the parking situation is beyond a joke. But four of our six patients were late to the hospital today for a combined tardiness of six hours! My favourite explanation was as follows: 'We had to wait two hours before we went to theatre after we arrived the last time, so we decided we'd just come two hours late today.'

There are many people who have to meet and review a patient before anyone proceeds for an operation: the admissions unit, the day ward secretary, the day ward nurses, the surgical team and the anaesthetist. There is good reason for this, as most people will understand. If you just got off the bus and simply walked into the nearest operating theatre to be anaesthetised, you may well end up with breast implants or a kidney transplant, that stubborn ingrown toenail you were hoping to have removed still throbbing as you wake up. *Enjoy your new breasts, Mr Murphy.* It's all about safety, assessing fitness for surgery and maximising the utility of our operating theatre resources. It's ok to be late, but please let us know if that is the case, so we can get another patient into theatre earlier.

Some delays, to be fair, are quite hilarious. Five-year-old Jack arrived in theatre today – very tentatively. He gingerly walked in, clinging to his father's leg, only to announce that he had to go to the toilet. Some pre-operative nerves no doubt, perfectly understandable. We point Dad in the direction of the toilet and off Jack scurries. Five minutes pass. No sign of little Jack. Ten minutes, nothing. I peer up the corridor to see Jack's dad still standing outside the toilet door. He gives me the scrunched-up face look and the 'so-so' see-saw hand gesture (think Gary Lineker gesturing to the bench in the 1990 World Cup semi-final as Gazza received a yellow card, ruling him out of the final) suggesting that things were going ok, but had not yet reached their epic conclusion. A full 16 minutes after Jack departed in a hurry, he came running back in, chirping triumphantly, 'Number 2, number 2, number 2!!' before hopping up onto the operating table, apparently a new man.

85 – Scoliosis

There are some 'major' subspecialties within paediatric anaesthesia that require a good deal of experience and regular practice. The more you practise something, the better and more comfortable you become at it. In my opinion, these include cardiac anaesthesia, airway anaesthesia, neonatal anaesthesia and scoliosis surgery. I am now three months into the job, found my footing on some of the more straightforward lists and am now ready to be tested further. Today I am listed to anaesthetise a child for major scoliosis surgery and tomorrow I will work on a major airway reconstruction case. It's a challenging week.

Scoliosis is a deformity of the spine. The spine is excessively curved and rotated, leaving a child with an uncomfortably hunched, twisted and disfiguring posture. It is associated with many congenital syndromes including muscular dystrophy, or can occur idiopathically (for no discernible reason) in otherwise healthy children. Sometimes surgical intervention is indicated. Surgery is offered not just for cosmetic reasons, but also to prevent or limit damage in other body systems. Unrepaired scoliosis can result in lung and heart dysfunction and even severe pain. Ideally, definitive surgery is deferred until after puberty, when the major growth spurt has finished. A major surgical correction can take all day and have a significant impact on the child, and thus it is a major surgical and anaesthetic challenge.

Straightening out a scoliotic spine can be hazardous surgery with significant blood loss. Even more seriously, it can leave a child either temporarily or permanently paralysed due to changes in the spinal cord itself. To prevent this, in every scoliosis operation neurophysiologists are present. They cover the patients in small electrodes all over the limbs and head. Throughout the surgery, and especially when the spine is being manipulated, they test the sensory and motor functions of the spinal cord to ensure it is still function-ing normally. As you can imagine, if an abnormal signal is detected, the surgeon must work quickly to find the root of the problem and correct it before permanent damage occurs. Communication between surgeon, neurophysiologist and anaesthetist is key.

On top of all this, to facilitate surgery on the spine, the child must be face down (prone). It is the anaesthetist's responsibility to ensure that the child is in a safe position to avoid any pressure injuries in this unnatural position. Pressure injuries in prone surgery can be as minor as a pressure blister on your knee or as serious as blindness due to excessive pressure on the eyes from poor position-ing. If we're uncomfortable in bed at night, we briefly awaken and shuffle into a new position, but clearly this isn't possible if you're under anaesthesia. Moreover, we cannot adjust the patient's posi-tion during surgery, so it is key to get it right from the beginning.

In one common operation to correct scoliosis, called a posterior spinal fusion, the surgeon exposes the entire spine, making an inci-sion from neck to pelvis. They dissect away the paraspinal muscles to expose the 'spinous processes', the bony prominences you can feel in the middle of your back. In a patient with scoliosis, they are not in a straight line, but curved in a 'c' or 's' shape. The exposed spinous processes almost make us look reptilian, like a dinosaur you might see in a museum. The surgeons then drill many precise holes into the vertebrae, using x-ray to determine the exact trajectory needed, and set screws in place. A rogue drill or misplaced screw, out of position by only a millimetre or two, could end up in the spinal canal itself. The final part of the surgery sees a long metal rod passed between the screws before being slowly tightened in place. As the rods are set, the spine is pulled into a straighter, more upright position.

Our patient today was a teenager, Sam, with idiopathic scoliosis. A nice case to begin my career in scoliosis surgery. The operation lasted eight hours from the time I put him to sleep to the time he woke up. You would be right in thinking that providing anaesthesia for one super-long operation could be boring. It can be, but sometimes we like boring. Today was good, and boring, and Sam leaves with a beautifully straight spine. His recovery will be tough, but our specialist orthopaedic nurses and physiotherapists will be helping Sam out of bed not even 24 hours after this major surgery.

86 – Surgical Doughnuts

The scoliosis operation I described yesterday is generally challenging as it is multi-faceted, long surgery where several things can go wrong. Today is challenging for another reason – relinquishing control. I'm certain that if you lined up a group of anaesthetists and sat them down to do a personality test we would all be diagnosed as anal-retentive control freaks with a mild caffeine addiction. But why, then, have I described myself, my colleagues and anaesthetists in general as being quite cool, calm and collected? Doesn't sound compatible with being controlling sociopaths, does it? But you can't have surgery without anaesthesia, so 99 per cent of the time we have the control of the operating room. We supply the oxygen, we keep the patient asleep, we decide if someone isn't suitable to be anaesthetised. Lots of things are on our terms. We are a bunch of big children who are used to getting our way. If we don't like what we see, we head home with the football so nobody else can play.[29]

Today the ENT surgeon is performing a laryngo-tracheal reconstruction (LTR). I'll do my best to describe what is going on here, just to give you some insight into why it is squirmy for the anaesthetist. When we breathe through our nose or mouth, the air passes through the voice box (larynx) into the windpipe (trachea) before reaching our lungs where the precious, life-preserving oxygen passes into the bloodstream. As you are all amateur anaesthetists by now, you will recall that when we render someone unconscious we place either a laryngeal mask airway (LMA) above the larynx or an ETT into the trachea, to assist with the supply of oxygen to the lungs. You know this better than you think, because without that oxygen stuff you'd be dead. Now picture this: there are a number of abnormalities of the larynx and trachea, some mild and some severe. Some are congenital and some acquired over time for various reasons. One type of iatrogenic (caused by medical interventions) abnormality is called 'subglottic stenosis',[30] a narrowing just below the vocal cords.

This can occur if a baby has had an ETT in place for a prolonged period of time because the tube irritates the inside of the trachea, leading to scarring, fibrosis and, ultimately, a severe narrowing when the ETT is finally removed. The effort of trying to breathe through a severely narrowed trachea is like going for a run while breathing through a straw. The babies breathe noisily, can get exhausted and even the slightest bit of additional swelling (from a

29 I may say we have 'control', but we proceed with 99 per cent of operations the surgeons need to do.

30 Short Latin lesson – *sub* = below, *glottis* = vocal cords (which are part of the larynx) and *stenosis* = narrowing.

cold or some phlegm) can be disastrous. Subglottic stenosis doesn't always need to be treated, but in severe cases a child might need a tracheostomy. This is a surgically placed tube in the lower trachea (below the stenosis) that allows the child to breathe with less effort and acts as a safety device.

A tracheostomy, however, doesn't fix the problem. If a child is to speak and breathe normally in future, the ENT surgeons have a number of operations up their sleeves to correct the stenosis. On the more severe and major end of this is the operation that we are performing today. Our child is a little girl called Lara, who already has a tracheostomy in place. The gist of the operation is that the surgeons slice open the trachea where the stenosis is situated, take some cartilage from the ribs and use it as a splinter device to open up the narrowing. This is done because parts of the larynx and trachea are also made of cartilage. Imagine slicing open a Dunkin Donuts doughnut on two opposite sides and inserting some pieces of a Krispy Kreme doughnut in the gaps you made to make a new doughnut with a larger hole in the middle. Easy.

Lara has been through this several times because unfortunately these efforts have thus far been unsuccessful. She has had a tracheostomy since she was an infant. She was born prematurely and had been intubated for prolonged periods early in life, resulting in her subglottic stenosis. With the tracheostomy in place and the narrowing above it, she cannot speak, and thus the surgeons are keen to have another attempt at fixing the problem. She is so familiar with the process of inducing anaesthesia that she immediately grabs the anaesthetic tubing out of my hand and attaches it directly to her tracheostomy, motioning at me to get on with it. She doesn't want to hear my rambling bollocks today. She falls asleep rapidly and we are ready to have attempt number four at reconstructing her trachea.

Where have I relinquished control, you might be asking? Well, because it's an operation on the trachea, we cannot place an ETT via the nose or mouth. As soon as she is asleep, our surgeon whips out the tracheostomy tube and makes a long incision above the orifice left behind in the trachea. The airway is completely exposed to the atmosphere and the child isn't breathing. Where we are used to cementing our ETT to the face or nose, such is the fear of it coming out, now our surgeon just nonchalantly places one in the far end of the trachea, headed towards the lungs. We attach the ventilator to the ETT so the lungs continue to do what they're supposed to, but he doesn't even bother to tape the ETT in place, as he knows it will be moved repeatedly throughout the operation. He has to do this to perform the operation. I can't get my controlling little hands anywhere near it. I have five hours of this to endure. When the ETT falls out (and it will, all day), I rely on the ENT surgeon to notice and also put it back in. Our anaesthetic ventilator will alarm if it is dislodged, but only after ten seconds or so. From where I am, I can't see what the surgeon is doing and my ventilator is alarming so much you would be forgiven for thinking it is having a seizure. Trust me, this is as squirmy as it gets for the anaesthetist. I picture the opposite: a surgeon turns around to find me with a scalpel in hand, preparing to make an incision in the aorta. I'm not sure many of them would remain conscious if they had to endure that.

Our ENT surgeons are well aware of the precarious state of affairs, though, and are superb communicators. The tube falls out so many times that by the end I don't even need to turn my head to the ventilator alarms as I know they will place the tube back correctly within seconds. I lost count, but I'd estimate it fell out or was removed intentionally around 30 times. That's 30 heart attacks for the surgeon watching an anaesthetist hack away around the aorta. The operation appears to be successful, but it is a long road to recovery. Lara will remain with a tracheostomy initially until we can see some improvement. She will go back to PICU and remain almost completely anaesthetised for several days after surgery to ensure she doesn't wake up and dislodge her precarious raw tracheostomy or any critical suture lines. I have faith, though – she is a tough kid.

92 – This Isn't a Hotel

Strange things patients do: Number 8374.

For some reason that is beyond me, a fairly low-risk child was admitted to the ward last night in preparation for a routine procedure today. Unless you are crocked to the point where a haircut may be a life-ending procedure for you, you do not require admission to the hospital before surgery. As it happened, I had arrived to meet them in the morning before anyone from the surgical team had the opportunity to obtain consent for the procedure. As I launched into my explanation of how I would anaesthetise their child, the parents stopped me in my tracks.

'We don't want him to have surgery.'

'Excuse me?'

'Yes. We've been thinking about it over the last few weeks and we decided we don't want him to have surgery.'

Well, I hope you enjoyed your stay at our hotel. The breakfast buffet is first class, isn't it?

I suggested that they wait to have a conversation with the surgeons about why the surgery was indicated and to discuss the risks. As I waited, the nurse on the ward told me that they had even expressed the same opinion when they arrived on the ward the night before. They didn't want surgery. *Seriously, what are they doing here?* The surgeons arrived and tried but sadly failed to convince them of the merits of the operation that was discussed and agreed upon in the outpatient clinic. The family headed off, delighted, after an uncomfortable and unnecessary night stay in a surgical ward, taking up a bed.

This phenomenon is not unique to paediatric practice; it occurs frequently in adult practice too. Patients turn up for appointments or even operations that they don't need any more. Before you think I sound a bit harsh, I will fully admit that our waiting lists for outpatient clinics or radiology appointments are ridiculously long. Comically long in fact. To the point that ailments that necessitated a referral in the first place may have resolved over time and patients genuinely have forgotten why they had been referred in the first place. Time heals all.

Well, what's the harm, I hear you say? Yes, it's true, some maniacs 'electrocuted' a man to death in Stanley Milgram's famous experiment on obeying authoritative figures, but when the price is inflicting unnecessary damage to yourself, you'd assume common sense would prevail. I've had patients turn up to have lumbar discs removed for pain they no longer had, colonoscopies for symptoms that disappeared months ago and now deciding against a perfectly straightforward procedure to prevent future pain for a child.

Anyway, what do I know, I'm just the guy who puts you to sleep. *Next!*

93 – St Patrick, Bank Official

I have popped out of theatre to grab a quick coffee between cases. The walk to the coffee shop takes me past the one and only ATM in the hospital. It's a temperamental, ageing machine with the 'out of service' screen featuring at least once a week. As I approach, a man stands at the machine looking a bit perplexed. He turns to see me in my blue scrubs and grabs my arm as I walk past.

'Sorry, do you work here?'

'Yes, I do.'

'Great. Listen, the ATM machine is after swallowing my card.'

'That's annoying.'

'Yeah. Can you sort it out for me?'

'Excuse me?'

'You must know how to get on to the bank or whatever?'

'I actually don't. I'm one of the doctors.'

'Fuck sake.'

I stroll away, perplexed by his expectation of a random man with a 'Batman' hat on his head. Bank official is far from the most bizarre thing I've been taken for. In Australia, they had me pegged for a snake-charmer. Yes, that's right, an Irishman was asked to catch a snake in a country full of snakes. Had they never heard of St Patrick? On that occasion, I was the only doctor in the emergency department of a small suburban hospital just outside Sydney. There were another couple of doctors on the wards and one in intensive care. It was a quiet night, and as I dozed with my head on the desk at 3 a.m., the phone rang.

'Did you say *snake*? In the storeroom?'

'Yes, in the children's ward,' replied the Australian nurse.

'Why are you calling me? Where are the other doctors? You do realise I'm Irish!'

'The other doctors are in surgery and won't be out for a while. The ICU doctor is busy. We have to call the most senior doctor when anything outside normal practice occurs.'

Fucking hell. How many things are wrong with those state-ments? One year qualified, I'm the most senior doctor available, from the land of *no snakes*, and am being asked to manage a snake in the land of deadly snakes. This must be a joke. I arrive up to the ward and the 6 foot 4 security guard is standing at the door of the store room. 'There's no way I'm going in there, mate!' he chuckled helpfully.

The head nurse stood at the door. She glared through the small glass window in the door and gestured at me to come and have a look. I peered through the window and, sure enough, on the shelves on the back wall hung the tail-end of a brown and black snake. Several other nurses stood guarding the doors of the kids on the ward, who were all asleep, awaiting the news on how I planned on catching the bastard. I couldn't see the head of the beast but there must have been half a metre of snake visible, dangling nonchalantly off the shelf.

'Guys, honestly, what do you expect me to do with this? I've never seen a snake in real life before.'

'You'll have to come up with a plan, though.'

'There is no way I am going in there, not a chance. There must be someone who deals with this.'

The head snake nurse and I headed to the computer as the security guard was tasked with watching the snake. A swift Google later and we had an out-of-hours state animal control service on the way. I ran back down to the emergency department to ensure everyone was ok and no one else had arrived. All clear (I don't think I've ever seen an empty emergency department in Ireland), so I slithered back up the stairs 20 minutes later just before the snake man arrived.

'Thank God you're here. We're lucky the thing hasn't moved yet.'

'Yeah no worries, mate. Where's the little troublemaker?'

The snake man picked up his bag and a long metal pole which I assumed was for him to pole vault out the window if the snake got too close. We scuttled behind him, glad of his reassuring presence. He sat the equipment down and strode over, looked in the little window for all of two seconds and opened the door confidently. As he strode inside, fearless, he glanced over at us. 'That's not a snake, mate. Not a chance,' he quipped. He walked straight to the back of the room and grabbed the tail of the terrifying and deadly monster. He pulled gently and out swung a brown and black snake. We took a step back, cowering. A scream rang out, maybe mine, I can't recall. Except the thing didn't move. There was no hiss. No fangs. There were no thrusting bites. It was a toy snake.

'Guys, no snake sits in a room this bright, with his tail there for all to see. Just so you know in future.'

And with that, the heroic snake man was gone with a story to tell all his other tough snake mates. The next step was to figure out which of the kids on the ward thought it would be hilarious to leave a toy snake in the storeroom. I didn't have time for the inquisition but was reliably informed that a sorrowful nine-year-old boy owned up to it the next morning.

Doctors: preservers of life, Hippocratic students, the wizened healers, retrievers of debit cards, and St Patrick, resurrected.

95 – Buzz for Entry

> 'Everyone remembers the day a dog
> ran into the school'
>
> – Peter Kay

It wasn't quite a dog today, but we had a very unexpected visitor in the MRI suite. It may be easier to break into Fort Knox or escape Alcatraz than to get into our MRI suite. There are three doors, all requiring swipe card access. To get a swipe card you must answer three riddles while juggling flaming hedgehogs. After this you must wrestle five knife-wielding ninjas to the death. The final door also requires a code which can only be won by simultaneously solving the Navier–Stokes equation and convincing Daenerys Targaryen to put her clothes back on.

This is mostly for safety reasons as, believe it or not, the MRI machine is incredibly dangerous if you go anywhere near it with metal objects. It is, after all, a giant, super-powered magnet. Imagine what Magneto could do with it? He'd probably reduce the waiting times, for one thing. Despite the obstacles required to get it, today we had an enormous bumblebee happily buzzing its way around the scanner; impressive, considering there are no open windows anywhere near the MRI suite. This lofty bee managed to prevail in his attempts to skip past our multiple security systems. On the other side of the corridor, the operating theatres are kept as clean as possible, for obvious reasons, but on very rare occasions a fly appears. If the staff are between cases, they can be seen flailing and flapping about in pursuit of the unsavoury character. If surgery is ongoing, often the anaesthetist goes on a solo mission. Evidently, I'm more comfortable dealing with small winged creatures than potentially poisonous snakes.

We feel bad trying to evacuate the bumblebee. But the valiant effort required to gain entry to the MRI suite has left him exhausted and he is not hard to catch. We have a quick multi-disciplinary team meeting and vote against euthanising him. I was ready with the anaesthetic gas to make it more humane than trampling on him. It was either that or ask the SHO to cannulate him. Our porter wraps him up and goes to find an open window. We can only assume the bee was on the non-urgent MRI waiting list and was just chancing his wing to get scanned today. Unfortunately, like everyone else, he will have to wait the mandatory 18 months before getting the MRI of his stinger.

98 – Work It

The following things make me squirmy and uncomfortable:

A knee being twisted in the wrong direction
Being too hot
Watching the *Titanic* sex scene with my parents
A child asking me to tell them a joke
Small talk

Our National Congress of Anaesthesia has been on in Dublin over the last couple of days. Every year, I look forward to it and, equally, want to avoid it all at the same time. I am perfectly comfortable in my own company. There are only a few people that I can spend long periods of time with (thankfully my wife is one of them).[31] I am a reasonable conversationalist in small groups of people I know well, but throw me into a larger social group or, worse, a networking event, and I can get uncomfortable very quickly. I was the child who wouldn't talk to kids I didn't know, would hide if there were guests in the house or wouldn't talk to my aunt on the phone who called to wish me a happy birthday. Being outgoing, suave and publicly entertaining was just never my thing. Complete strangers are the worst for me as I tend to be someone who observes group dynamics and personalities from a safe distance before coming out of my shell. Throw me in with a complete stranger and I squirm when I'm talking about the weather for lack of a better topic. Maybe that's why I'm a good anaesthetist: I'll just put you to sleep before the small talk commences. *Tell me more about your cats (*grabs large syringe of propofol*).*

Medical conferences are much like any other conference – there are a series of sessions on various subjects, in various rooms over the course of a couple of days. In between we drink weak coffee and industry salespeople try to sell us things we don't need or can't afford. It's as much a social event as an educational event. International speakers are invited to speak and Irish anaesthetists working abroad will return to attend. From a social perspective, it's nice to meet up with peers whom I haven't seen in a while. I count my lucky stars that I have a consultant post already, as I see others 'working the room'. It has to be done. They have to make sure that senior anaesthetists in a particular hospital remember them, to let them know you'll be applying for any upcoming consultant jobs. Smile and nod. Talk about the weather. *How are the kids?* It's so competitive. I hide in the corner with a couple of close friends.

What is evident from medical conferences is that if you ever think you're on top of your game and a world-leading expert, there

---

31 Not out of dislike for anyone, just a preference for some peace and quiet.

is always someone more accomplished than you. I greatly admire doctors who carry out medical research. It is extremely time-consuming, expensive and occasionally infuriating. Yet there are some who manage to persevere, and they change medical practice and improve patient outcomes through that sheer grit and determination. There are several world-renowned professors at the conference this year. They all appear to be great pals, but I wonder deep down do they actually all hate each other?

'Oh, you published in *The New England Journal of Medicine* last month? Great!' *Teeth grinding*

Two statistics that get mentioned as professors are introduced before taking to the podium to deliver a lecture are: a) how many journal publications they have; and b) how much money they have received in research grants. Think Instagram likes and penis length. '*Professor X has 900 publications and received $30 million in grants.*' Professor X also has a full-time clinical job, volunteers at the homeless shelter, has four beautiful children, is editor of six journals, has written three books, co-wrote 'Every Breath You Take' with Sting, won gold in the high jump at the Sydney Olympics in 2000, is vegan and climbed Mount Everest blindfolded. *What do you mean you've never been up Everest?* Where do they all find the time?

For the record, my publication count is *huge*.

99 – Inception

Now I've managed to come this far into my musings and not really mentioned the superheroes of any hospital – the nursing staff. We rely so heavily on the nursing staff that I'll be honest, I'm slightly concerned that they could make my life hell if they don't like what I write about them. So let me start with the fact that they are the hardest-working and most underappreciated group in any hospital.[32]

---

32 This was not written under duress. I promise.

What I admire most in the nursing staff is their organisational skills. When a nurse reaches management level, be it in theatre, the wards or elsewhere, they become clinical nurse managers (CNM). Every individual operating theatre has one or two CNMs that manage the throughput of that theatre on a given day. Experienced CNMs run a tight ship; *they* are the real bosses in theatre – forget about the surgeon or the anaesthetist.

Yet a quality CNM makes every surgeon or anaesthetist think that they are calling the shots. A CNM can bore deep into my subconscious, plant a few little seedlings and wait for them to sprout branches out of my own gob. As ideas bubble into my consciousness, I pat myself on the back, impressed with my logistical prowess, completely unaware that the CNM has planted these plans hours ago. 'That's a great idea, Colin.' If you've ever seen *Inception*, you'll know what I mean. Alas, we are merely memetic vectors for the CNMs' plans. Generally, they have more experience working with a particular surgeon than I have, so they know what delays to expect, where we might encounter equipment issues and what operations the surgeon might be better off performing in the morning or afternoon.

Typically, their skill comes in organising the order of the operating list. While generally speaking we like to do either tiny babies or day-case surgery first in the morning, inevitably, the CNM has already been talking to the day unit, or intensive care, knows where the surgeons are and how many nursing staff they have at their disposal for the day. The CNM knows what patient is ready to go, what patient hasn't turned up yet, what patient needs the surgeons to gain consent, what patient needs anaesthetic review, what patient has been given something to drink while they wait, whether the surgeon is in the building, what colour underpants I am wearing or even what the surgical SHO had for breakfast. Where I might make a suggestion on how we proceed, I am nearly always overruled, but not in a confrontational way; the CNM is very subtle. I let them do their thing in managing the flow, and try to take a passive approach, to be flexible. That way, if there is something I feel strongly about, when I do pipe up, then I'm more likely to be heard. It's one area where I'm happy to relinquish control and focus on other tasks.

A real challenge for any CNM is the emergency list. The tricky thing with the emergency list is the simultaneous juggling of surgeons from many different specialties trying to get cases into the emergency theatre, maximising the limited theatre time and ensuring the staff get home on time. The frustrating thing about the emergency list is the very fact that the cases are emergencies. They are not scheduled, elective operations, so inevitably there are delays: the patient isn't ready, the patient hasn't been fasting for long enough, or the required surgeon isn't available at that very moment. But the CNM juggles all these flaming batons without much trouble.

I had notions about myself this morning, thinking I knew exactly how the emergency list would run. We had four cases listed in the morning, but this had ballooned to ten by 10 a.m. We make a reasonable start but, at least an hour before I realise it, our CNM knew we wouldn't get all the cases done by 6 p.m. So, she has already offloaded two cases to other theatres, convinced a surgeon that one can wait until tomorrow, fashioned a spare surgical registrar out of thin air and now has acquired me a second theatre in which to work.

'Colin, the appendicectomy has just gone into Theatre 2 and the fracture has gone into Theatre 4. You better start the fracture first because the child is only four. Your reg can start the appendix. We need to get cracking to finish by six.'

I get in there and I bloody get started as soon as possible. We finish just about on time.

Other than keeping the show on the road, the CNMs also have to act as advocates for the nursing staff. Most surgeons would operate late if they were allowed to. They would love nothing more than to be immersed in a sea of urine or lost in a forest of colon; their happy place. So it takes a brave person to say 'no' on occasion. The nursing staff regularly stay beyond their rostered working hours, so if a CNM stands their ground when a surgeon wants to push on and operate late, it is greatly appreciated by their junior colleagues (and, quite frankly, by me too).

100 – Trust

Children are such diverse and unpredictable creatures. At one end of the spectrum you have kids who run into the hospital with glee to visit the nurses and the giant fish tank in the corridor. Sometimes they're even looking forward to seeing their favourite doctor. At the other end, just the idea of having to go to the hospital can terrify a child. The latter group can include both the 'frequent fliers' who regularly attend the hospital or complete newbies who have never even been to a hospital. Beyond fear of the unknown, I have often wondered what it is that makes new attendees afraid of the hospital. I think a lot of cues come from parental attitudes to the hospital. When we are anaesthetising children, the anxious kids often have anxious parents who are tearful on the trip into the operating theatre. On the contrary, the children who fly through their anaesthetic often have parents who are nonchalant about the whole thing. There is a sweet spot somewhere.

But kids aren't stupid. No, it might not have been a great idea to attempt to draw Sponge Bob on your newly painted kitchen wall. No, the dog probably didn't need to wear your mother's lipstick. And no, it wasn't the best idea to empty all the bean bags and roll around in them naked (hats off to a four-year-old me and my two-year-old sister for that one). But children definitely have a sixth sense of knowing when something is not quite right, even those without the vocabulary to tell you. The child who is normally at ease can become uptight when encountering a new environment. Or a child who is already uptight can become hysterical.

The story of our patient today has some negatives and some positives. Diarmuid attended with his father to have a procedure on a narrowing of his aorta. The procedure was not via open surgery, but via a catheter inserted into the blood vessels in his groin by the cardiologist: a minimally invasive procedure with good results. Diarmuid had been to his GP recently with abdominal pain and the astute GP listened for his heart sounds and diagnosed a murmur which turned out to be a coarctation of the aorta.[33] A superb diagnosis, seeing as this is usually picked up in much smaller children.

The trouble began when Diarmuid arrived in the day ward. The cardiology registrar attended to explain the procedure and gain consent from his parents. This was the first time he had heard that a) he had a problem with his aorta and b) he was in hospital to be anaesthetised and have it corrected – today. This news was followed by hysteria, tears and fear so intense that it led to vomiting and retching. I arrived about 15 minutes later to see the poor lad quivering in his room, livid with his dad for misleading him. He was under the impression he was here for an x-ray to investigate further the abdominal pain. It is hard for all of us, nursing and medical staff, to turn around a situation like this, especially when a child is old enough to comprehend their well-being and a medical procedure. It is not uncommon to have children arrive in theatre with only a vague idea of why they're there, with parents instructing us to just 'get on with it'.

As soon as children are old enough to ask sensible questions about their bodies and health, they have a right to know what's going on. As anaesthetists, we can't just 'get on with it' as the

---

33 A murmur is the sound of turbulent blood flow inside the heart or a blood vessel usually as a result of a 'hole' between two chambers of the heart, damaged heart valves or other abnormal strictures in blood vessels.

process of being anaesthetised could be perceived by the child as little short of an assault on them. While they may not be able to legally consent to the operation itself, they must have some understanding as to why they need to be anaesthetised and comply with us. For obvious reasons, this is not possible with small infants and toddlers. Compliance with anaesthesia starts long before we even set eyes on a child. When the decision is made that an operation is required, that is when children need to have some mental preparation for what lies ahead. It's just not fair to be sprung with a major life event mere moments before it begins. The stepping stone to this particular life event is anaesthesia, and this is often where the most apprehension lies. For major operations, there are child psychologists who specialise in preparing children for surgery. There are some occasions when, despite fantastic preparation, a child is still super-anxious. In these scenarios, we can administer a premedication that can alleviate some of the anxiety. These can work beautifully, but can result in kids that (sometimes hilariously) appear at advanced levels of inebriation – possibly a glimpse into their university years ahead.

With help from the nursing staff and a play specialist, we managed to alleviate some of Diarmuid's angst. A positive. I was able to answer his questions about anaesthesia (of which there were many). His retching stopped. We discussed a premedication, which he agreed to and took himself. After around 30 minutes he appeared relaxed enough to come to theatre. There were a few more tears on the way, but nothing quite like earlier in the morning. He was compliant with anaesthesia and the procedure was straightforward.

Children like to have a certain degree of control and independence once they reach a critical age, and any dent in this perceived control can result in frustration and mistrust that can be hard to regain. It is crucial to manage a child's expectations. They need to know they're going to the hospital. They need to know they're having an operation. They need to hear how they will be anaesthetised. I try to talk to them like they're teenagers, or adults, if appropriate.

Although he skipped out of hospital later that afternoon, I can't help but think it will take Diarmuid time to build up trust with his parents again.

102 – Michelin Babies

As I listened to the radio on my drive home today I was surprised to learn that 'fat shaming' is now the most common form of childhood bullying. It has surpassed height, glasses-wearing, ethnicity or questions of sexuality as the most common reason for kids to be picked on. Is it a coincidence that I anaesthetised an older boy who weighed over 100 kilograms today? That is far from the heaviest child requiring anaesthesia in our department recently; one young patient just last week topped out at 120 kg.

I was never bullied in school, but even being picked on (mostly in jest, I hope) about my monobrow certainly made me feel self-conscious. If I was returning any slagging, all my jousting opponent would have to do was raise a single finger across the breadth of their two eyebrows, indicating my monobrow, to make my blood boil. But at least I could go home and pluck the caterpillar out from between my eyes. *But what if they slag me more because I plucked it out?! Then they'll know they got to me!* Oh, the woes of secondary school.[34]

I have mixed feelings about the subject of obesity. On the one hand, I have such sympathy for anyone who is bullied in school. Kids can be so cruel. Being bullied for being overweight is compounded by the fact that you can't change overnight, and even

---

34 For the record, I only plucked it out in university, and it requires ongoing maintenance on an almost daily basis.

if you work at it for months, kids have long and scarily accurate memories. It's a label you're often stuck with. From the medical perspective, though, obesity is a rampant epidemic with serious adverse health effects for both children and adults. There are a very small number of medical conditions and a very small number of medications that can cause weight gain. Weight gain is really quite simple – if your caloric intake is greater than your caloric expenditure, you will gain weight. This is a long-term phenomenon, consistency over time. The two pieces of cake you ate at the birthday party will not make you fat, but two pieces of cake per day is an issue. It sounds simple, but it's not as simple as that.

Unfortunately, we are starting to see obesity from an even younger age now too. While we see many chubby babies, they 'grow out' of their padding once they become mobile and start expending calories by crawling. But there is an increasing number of toddlers and children under the age of eight who are obese. On some occasions, I have had to get an ultrasound machine out to help me cannulate a vein, such is the depth of the fat we are trying to work around.

Yes, a consistent caloric surplus will result in weight gain, but do we do enough as doctors, nutritionists, educationalists, public health professionals or social service professionals to provide, not only the ability to obtain nutritious food, but the tools to prepare it? It is no secret that there is a socioeconomic class division in obesity rates. Children take their nutrition cues from their parents; they can't eat what they're not given. But some children with learning difficulty or behavioural problems won't settle unless they get the food they like. Nutritious, fresh food is expensive and not to everyone's taste. Preparing delicious healthy meals is hard if you are coming off the back of a long day at work and have never been taught how to do so. It is easier and cheaper to open a bag of Doritos.

It's hard to hear, but the changes required to tackle childhood obesity start with tackling adult obesity.

105 – One Shot of Adrenalin Please, Sir

The airline industry is often compared to anaesthesia when it comes to safety. The similarities were noted by an airline pilot whose wife, Elaine Bromiley, unexpectedly and tragically died during induction of anaesthesia.[35] In the inquiry into the incident many human factors were flagged as contributing to the death. Ms Bromiley's husband has since been a leading proponent of human factors in clinical errors which has led to many important practice changes, not only within anaesthesia.

The analogy, to be fair, is a nice one. An airline pilot and co-pilots go through a series of checks to ensure everything is in order before taking off. They go through specified processes and check-lists for everything. This ensures they safely make the plane airborne, they then keep the plane cruising in the sky, before a safe and controlled descent results in a successful landing. The anaesthetist and team learn the patient's history and makes a plan for surgery. We then induce anaesthesia (take-off), maintain anaesthesia and make small adjustments during surgery (cruising at altitude) before allowing a controlled emergence from anaesthesia at the end of surgery (landing). However, the analogy is now such a cliché to anaesthetists that any mention of the airline industry is met with groans as eyes roll to heaven.

Where the analogy falls down, however, is that sometimes anaesthesia is not always as smooth as expected and circumstances dynamically change during surgery. Where a Boeing 737 is always

---

35 'Induction' is the process of placing a patient into a state of general anaesthesia: 'I induce anaesthesia.' Induction of anaesthesia is achieved using either intravenous drugs or inhaled gases. Following 'induction' there is 'maintenance' of anaesthesia. Again, maintenance can be achieved by continuous intravenous infusion of drugs or continuous delivery of volatile anaesthetic gases. Once the surgery is completed, the anaesthesia agent of choice is discontinued, and the patient is allowed to wake up – this is 'emergence'.

going to be a Boeing 737, not every patient is the same. Try taking off when both your wings are on fire. Try staying on your planned flight path when the Luftwaffe are unloading on your engine. Try landing the plane at night with no lights on the runway. It's sometimes a lot harder than we give ourselves credit for. From a personal perspective, I felt I had almost reached cruising altitude over the last three months. Until today, when the engines were set on fire during induction of anaesthesia.

A toddler with a complex medical background appeared for a relatively minor procedure. Despite this, I expected him to be straightforward to anaesthetise. Fast forward to five minutes later, with the child partially anaesthetised, there was little to no oxygen being transmitted to his gas-exchanging alveoli. His mid-sized airways, the bronchi, appeared to be in spasm. We call this a bronchospasm. To make things worse, he added a large vomit just to make sure my bowels were paying attention. My adrenal glands fired out a healthy dose of their adrenalin special brew for my heart to taste. I questioned why I was being so sadistic to myself? Is this enjoyable? *I could just work for Facebook and sit on a beanbag, sipping americanos, brainstorming about the next Internet fad. I could open a bar on a beach in Thailand. Wouldn't it be nice to run a small B&B in rural West Cork?* Thankfully, these fleeting thoughts only occurred to me after the alarm bell rang and the situation was rectified with the rapid help of some of my skilled colleagues.

In fact, this is the thing that is so appealing for me in paediatric anaesthesia: the expected, unexpected events that keep me on my toes and keeps the job interesting. What sort of self-loathing individuals enjoy the rush of adrenalin and cognitive stress that comes on an almost regular basis? Paediatric anaesthetists and paediatric intensive care doctors, that's who! I don't wish terror on myself, but the *prospect* of terror really makes me concentrate in work and keeps the brain engaged at all times. I think some of the appeal is working in an area that frightens the life out of other anaesthetists. Do we have a superiority complex? Are we adrenalin junkies? I really don't think so. Perhaps I'm more scared about being bored in a career that lasts a lifetime. I think I'll accept my monthly adrenalin shot.

106 – Alice

I don't know how many people work in the operating theatre department and intensive care, but I'd estimate it's about 17,000,000. At least, that's what it feels like when you move to a new hospital. Operating departments are huge, populated with doctors and surgeons, nurses of all kinds (managers, scrub, circulating, anaesthesia, recovery, day ward, intensive care, pain), healthcare assistants, perfusionists, porters, medical engineers, cleaning staff, receptionists and secretaries. There are just so many faces and names to learn. I recognise faces very well. I can tell you where I met someone before, easy. *He was mean to me in primary school. I kissed her in a disco when I was 15. She walks her dog near our house. He shot JR.* But learning and remembering names is, for some reason, the black hole of my memory bank. It is a very slow, tortuous and challenging venture for me. It really is amazing how fast a name escapes my brain. It literally takes seconds.

'Colin, this is Sarah.'

'Hi, Sarah, how are you getting on? What department do you work in?'

'I'm one of the intensive care nurses.'

What the fuck is this person's name ... think ... Sally? No. Shit. Where's her name badge ...

I have worked in this very hospital before, so many names have come back to me easily enough, but the staff turnover in hospitals is a lot higher than one might expect, especially for nursing staff. Nurses may decide to move out of theatre to the wards, or more often move abroad for lifestyle or work experience. The new faces and new names are taking their time to settle in.

We have a very small tearoom where everyone crams in to eat lunch and drink coffee on their breaks. Some days it's like a night-club, squeezing past people to get to the microwave, drinks being spilled. It always feels slightly warmer than you're comfortable with as the afternoon sun soaks the room to top up the stuffy heat of the radiator that seems to have been stuck in the 'on' position for the last six years. There is a single telephone in the corner which rings frequently, usually looking for a specific person to come up to a specific operating theatre. I foolishly took the decision to answer the phone today, breaking one of my cardinal rules: 'Never answer the phone unless you know all the names in the room.'

'No, sorry, Alice isn't here.'

A woman approached and took the receiver from me as I moved to put it down.

'I think that's for me.'

109 – Hungry Dogs

Ivan Pavlov managed to turn a previously neutral stimulus (a metro-nome) into a conditioned stimulus that eventually provoked a condi-tioned response (salivation). The metronome indicated that food was arriving, but after a short time the dogs would salivate on cue after the metronome, even if no food arrived. Although his experiments were carried out on dogs, I too am a mammal and possibly only slightly smarter than one of his hungry canine companions.

After my extremely difficult case in my first week on the job, the specific diagnosis we were dealing with on that day (a previously neutral stimulus) has resulted in surging levels of cortisol and adrenalin traversing my venous plexus (my conditioned response). After my rough experience, the mention of this diagnosis by colleagues has me thinking back to the day and what I could have done better. All with a side serving of sweaty palms and a slightly increased heart rate. But I think this conditioned response has served me well as today I am anaesthetising another neonate for the same problem.

Any surgery in neonates should raise the heart rate a little as the stakes are high and your best performance is required. I used to get butterflies in my stomach before a big sporting occasion, but I grew to learn that this meant I was focused, prepared and expecting a battle. Some of my best performances on a pitch came after feeling truly awful before a game. When I saw the case listed for theatre today, I got mildly anxious, but mostly very excited. I was prepared like it was a cup final. I considered wearing a three-piece suit and a boutonniere to work, as if I would soon be walking into Wembley stadium for the FA Cup final. I evaluated the opposition (the baby), predicted what performance they might put in (based on her comorbidities) and tailored my tactics around the scenario to ensure I would win the match this time.

When you ruminate over things over a period of time, it can sometimes be therapeutic. This time around, I had a clear plan in my head and visualised everything: the first pass, the first tackle, the first sprint. I talked everything through with my registrar – this is how we'll approach this, this is how we beat this baby (we don't *actually* beat the babies, but you know what I mean). The baby arrives. She is Lionel Messi, I am Richard Dunne. She is Goliath, I am David. But experience breeds confidence in anaesthesia. I have been here before – I know what worked and what didn't last time out. We have made well-thought-out tactical changes, fresh off the whiteboard in the training ground.

It was a clean sheet for Richard Dunne, a phenomenal performance. But this is not a zero-sum game. It might feel like a battle, but we are all really on the same team. I see myself as a facilitator for the baby to battle to victory and come through the operation. A win for us is also a win for the baby.

112 – 'The last desperate fart of a dying corpse'

Two or three times per week, a consultant will conduct a morning teaching session for our trainees. Any consultant who works in a university hospital has an obligation to provide teaching of some description, be it to undergraduate medical students or qualified doctors within their field of expertise. Every consultant in our department has their own area of interest. Some skillsets overlap, but you can usually wiggle yourself into a seat at the teaching table. Unfortunately for me, I'm the newest recruit to the department and there appears to be little room at the grown-ups' table. I'm sitting at the kids' table, eating fish fingers and beans. My particularly favourite area, cardiac anaesthesia, happens also to be many other consultants' favourite area and thus most of the teaching topics have been covered by others.

I sent my list of prepared lectures to my colleague who schedules the teaching: the history of cardiac surgery, blood clotting in cardiac surgery, monitoring in cardiac surgery, heart transplants, my top ten favourite things about the heart, total eclipse of the heart, I heart the heart. 'Sorry, Colin, we have all those covered.' *Sigh ... how about statistics?* I am no more a statistician than the Leaving Cert student interpreting the results of the SurveyMonkey they sent their pals on where they should go on holidays in the summer (Hersonissos, obviously). I'm not even convinced that statisticians enjoy statistics.

Nevertheless, here I am this morning with a lecture entitled 'P-values and Z Scores: Making Statistics Fun!' More like *zzzzzzz* scores. It does not begin well as there are only two people in the room at 7.45 a.m. Apparently my lecture wasn't on the teaching schedule. Anyone arriving even one minute late to this would do better going to a lecture on particle physics given in ancient Hebrew. Secondly, the ageing computer in the conference room hasn't got the latest version of PowerPoint, so there goes the safety net of the 'presenter view' and the ability to glance at my notes. So, at the moment we have two poor souls about to hear me attempting to recall my basic statistics module from 2013. Five minutes later, after a few WhatsApp messages, we have a quorum, so I begin.

The first head in the audience begins to bob after about six minutes, the second a minute later. Carl Friedrich Gauss would be appalled to see his work being disrespected so much. Maybe these two trainees were on night shift. I'll cut them some slack. It occurred to me that all those times I thought I was nodding off in a lecture room incognito, I was actually partially breaking the heart of someone who had put a lot of work into a lecture. If you're reading, I'm sorry. But there are a few interested faces, I'm surprised to see. Naturally, they will be receiving all of the eye contact. *Oh, I'm not letting you fall asleep, sir. Stay tuned for questions!* Most of the faces, however, are puzzled, like a baby who screws up their face, unsure if they're hungry, tired or about to destroy another nappy. The lecture peters out to a close, like, to borrow a phrase from Thom Yorke, 'the last desperate fart of a dying corpse'.

There were a few genuine 'thank yous' thrown my way, but these were followed by: 'I heard someone else use a fantastic analogy to explain all that before. He made it sound so easy ...' *Thanks?*

114 – Date Night

I'm off work tomorrow and a glance at the day's operating list suggests that we should be finished on time, by 5 p.m. I decide I should use the opportunity to take the two-hour journey west after work, to see my wife who still lives in Galway. One of the perks of two hospital doctors being in a relationship is that you get to live in separate cities for years on end. I tell her the good news. I should be in Galway by 7.30 p.m., so we make plans for dinner at 8 p.m. A rare date.

Our list starts well, and we get through the bulk of the work by 1 p.m. All that is left is the 'big case'. Getting stuck into the 'big case' by 1 p.m. is pretty good on most days. When the operator turns to me about 30 minutes in and says, 'This could take a while,' that's when the concern creeps in. Three o'clock rolls around and I hear, 'This could take another three or four hours.' *Ooooof*, like a blow to the stomach.

I'll never get stroppy with a surgeon – it's not like they always want to be there late into the evening, away from their own family either. We simply have a duty to the child who is anaesthetised on the table to get the job done as best we can, no matter how long it takes. Operations have been known to go on *all night*. It felt like all the heart transplants I worked on in London happened in the middle of the night. I'm fortunate that my wife is a surgeon, as I don't need to offer any explanation other than, 'I'm stuck in theatre, won't be there until late.' I imagine personal relationships can be difficult where one partner doesn't understand the acuity of some of the work in a hospital. You can't simply leave a patient.

By the time I arrive in Galway at 10.15 p.m., a sandwich and an episode of *Game of Thrones* will certainly suffice when it's been two weeks since I've seen my wife.

121 – Mixed Messages

I was impressed this afternoon to see parents taking photos of some of the information we have posted about sugar consumption in children. We have posters around the hospital indicating what the maximum healthy daily allowance of sugar is for children across all age ranges. One of the displays shows, for example, a can of Coca-Cola and beside it, in a small plastic bag, the corresponding raw sugar that it contains. The comparison is certainly eye-opening.

Despite how much effort goes into public health campaigns, the message about sugar is often missed by the public, no doubt because sugar is such an easy way to placate a child. In fact, we do it ourselves as medics when we give babies their soother dipped in sucrose before a painful procedure like an IV cannula. Desperate times …

But, in more normal circumstances, I was reassured to see some parents really taking it in, giving me some hope that our public health efforts aren't entirely in vain.

Fifteen minutes later, I saw the same parents smoking outside the hospital with their child in the buggy.

126 – Flushing Meadows

I want to talk about bladder capacity. As my wife is a urologist, I probably possess an above-average knowledge of the urinary system. Our dinner-table conversation, mostly via Facetime these days, usually touches on some of the following: techniques for shoving urinary catheters into bladders, the unique ability urologists have for determining weight by poking (the prostate), how priapism (a sustained, sometimes painful, erection) might actually be welcome if you're over 70 years of age, the largest penis she's ever seen, how many rectums she's had her finger in that day and why coffee makes you dying for a pee even if it's a small volume (it's a bladder irritant, apparently).

Urinating (volume, frequency, stream, colour and more) is fascinating to the urologist and I have learned that there is a lot of psychology involved in controlling one's bladder. For example, those who tend to 'need' to go a lot can often retrain this frequent sensation to pee by peeing at increasingly longer predetermined intervals. The phrase 'to piss oneself with fright' is a legitimate neurobiological response to catecholamines (e.g. adrenalin) that are released when you are scared. Some unfortunate people who suffer from urinary incontinence often have their day completely consumed by planning where the nearest toilet is.

I have come to realise that surgeons are bladder masters: they have tamed Pisseidon. As anaesthetists, there are usually two of us assigned to an operating theatre – a consultant and a trainee. Therefore, we have the luxury of heading off for a pee whenever the hell we want, and all the coffee we consume ensures that this is multiple times in a day. Surgeons, however, *never* seem to need to pee. They could stand there all day and all night and not complain, even for a second. The same goes for the scrub nurses who assist the surgeon, although their colleagues can mercifully bail them out to head to Flushing Meadows.

Our operation today took 11 hours. The surgeons were scrubbed in for ten of those hours. Even after they were finished, they remained in the operating room while we organised the patient for transfer and brought the child to intensive care. They didn't leave once. I, on the other hand, had three or four leisurely stops in the bathroom throughout the day. I assume my registrar had the same number – I stopped short of asking him if he went to the toilet on his break. So rare is it that I can remember the one time I got stuck in theatre dying for a pee. I had my head stuck out in the corridor desperately begging for someone to find *any* other anaesthetist to come and let me out for two minutes. It was hell. How do surgeons do this?

There are tactics involved. Surgeons are rarely seen gulping large pints of water in the tearoom, whereas part of the standard uniform of an anaesthetist is a trendy stainless steel or solid plastic water bottle from which we continually sip. I do worry about the health of our surgeons' poor kidneys. The intensive care unit is obsessed with urine output, as it is a useful indicator to how well your kidneys are working, especially when you're very sick. A study written (partially in jest) in 2010 suggested that doctors working in intensive care were more at risk of kidney injury than the patients they were caring for. The authors compared the urine output of the patients in intensive care with that of the doctors on shift. Spoiler alert: the doctors made less urine.[36]

Of all the different types of medicine one can train in, surgeons have the most all-consuming job. I don't mean that they are the busiest, but when they are operating they think of nothing else. It is pure, unadulterated focus – which is reassuring. As you can probably guess from the fact you are reading this book, I can muse and ponder life for large chunks of the day when we have patients settled in long surgery.

127 – Deceiving Appearances

I am lucky that I, so far, am in good health. I have no chronic illnesses bar the inevitable orthopaedic ailments that curse someone who had a fairly intense sports career. *Remember when my back didn't hurt?* The latest I'm contending with is plantar fasciitis which I can assure you is like someone prodding the sole of your foot with a hot poker with every ginger step. Oh my, those first few steps in the morning! But I wouldn't swap my minor inconveniences for any chronic illness – not eczema, not inflammatory bowel disease, arthritis or vasculitis.

Before I started working with children, I didn't really understand why everyone looked so relieved when their newborn was deemed to be healthy. *Weren't all babies healthy?* It's only when I started working in an environment where the concentration of sick children is obviously 1,000 times that of a local neighbourhood that I learned that it truly is a blessing/accident when a child is born in good health. In some instances, it is obvious when a child is unwell. They may have a distinctive appearance common to a particular syndrome, they may be scrawny or they may just have that washed-

---

36 BMJ 2010;341:c6761.

out look that comes from being drained by an underlying disease. But some sick kids appear quite well from the outside.

Today we anaesthetised several children with cystic fibrosis (CF), a genetic disease that affects the lungs most obviously, but also the gut, pancreas and kidneys. It is particularly common in Ireland due to our genetic fingerprint, and we screen for it at birth for this reason. People with CF often suffer from recurrent chest infections as they produce thick, sticky mucus that is hard to clear from the lungs. They often become colonised with particularly nasty pathogenic bacteria. Our list of cases today consisted solely of children with CF having their annual bronchoscopy to see exactly what bacteria are present deep in the lungs.[37] This, as always, involves a general anaesthetic.

Many of you will know a teenager or adult who suffers from CF. By the time they reach adulthood, you will usually notice they can be of short stature due to the chronicity of the disease and trouble absorbing essential nutrients from their diet. But the group of kids we anaesthetised today appeared, from the outside, to be entirely normal. Granted, they were very young children, so growth problems may not have been evident just yet.

Seeing this group today gave me pause for thought. Firstly, how good health and genetics are basically the opposite of the lottery. Most people win, but a small number don't. It isn't fair to be struck with a chronic disease from birth, having lost the genetic lottery. Secondly, one should never make assumptions about someone's health just because they 'look healthy'. That colleague who is frequently off work, that friend who never turns up for football or that 'lucky' girl who wears a size 0 may be contending with a lot more than you think.

---

37 The suffix '-oscopy' essentially means 'having an 'aul look at' with a camera. Bronchoscopy – having a look at the lungs. Colonoscopy – having a look at the colon. Laparoscopy – having a look inside the abdomen. You get the idea.

Although, sometimes people are just lazy bastards who don't show up for football.

128 – A Tale of Two Halves

Medical training does not cover many of the skills essential to the job. Yes, we have some professionalism courses that try to ensure you don't call someone a 'fuckwit' if they disagree with you, but these models of conflict resolution only really work if both parties are being reasonable. The subordinate trainees are not privy to the side-room discussions about many key decisions. But I have now been thrust into these scenarios with a flaming sheet of toilet paper stuffed down the back of my scrubs. I thought it was all roses, holding hands and smiley faces, but there is a lot more conflict that I anticipated.

As a consultant, I am now a gatekeeper of sorts. I can agree or refuse to anaesthetise a patient based on my opinion. I do my best to avoid confrontation, but I had to, for the first time, stand my ground on a matter regarding an extremely sick child. I refused to take a child to theatre on the grounds of futility. Regardless of whether we proceeded with a risky transfer to theatre from PICU for another procedure, the child would most likely die. I generally facilitate everyone to the best of my ability and I don't say no to cases very often.

It's tricky when I have been a subordinate not so long ago in this same hospital. It can take time for established consultants and other senior staff to view new consultants as peers and it's not comfortable disagreeing with a mentor. It's never personal, but simply two people advocating differing things, for the same patient. I felt under an uncomfortable amount of pressure to proceed with the case and I almost did. I felt awful, but I had to go with my gut instinct. A third and fourth consultant were drafted in to listen to our respective reasoning. They agreed with me. Although this went some distance to justifying my position, it didn't make me feel any different or victorious. I respect the person I had a disagreement with and have massive respect for their opinion.

Regardless of who 'won' the argument, we still had a terminally sick child, which doesn't put any gloss on the situation in the end.

130 – What's in a Name?

I thought I was bad with names, but I have met my match. There is a man who has a locker two down from mine in the changing rooms. Let's call him 'Peter'. Every day that I see Peter, I greet him by his name. 'Morning, Peter. How are things?'

The reply is always the same: 'Morning, yes. Hi, mumble, mumble.' Occasionally he attempts my name.

'Morning, Peter. How are things?'

'Fine, fine. How are you, Chris?'

About three seconds after I've walked past, and he's got my name wrong again, I hear a whispered 'Colin!' that chases me down the corridor.

Most of the time I bear witness to a look of fear topped with a dollop of confusion as I approach him. He knows I'm going to call him by his name. He knows he's forgotten mine, again. If we were on the street, he'd cross the road. But we're in the theatre corridor and our courses are set for an embarrassing collision. Next stop, mortification. I sometimes slow down so I can give him an extra second to think about it. Either that, or I give him an extra second of that squirmy feeling deep in the pit of his stomach. Peter sees my name in print at least three times in our daily transaction. On my ID card, on the name badge on my scrubs and, most obviously, on the locker he sees me opening every single morning. Perhaps this is the little piece of entertainment I keep to myself on a daily basis, just to break up the intensity of the job.

I have noticed one of our registrars doing the same thing, this time involving the staff in the café. He has noticed that every day, despite a soup being on the menu, no one has a clue what type of the soup they are actually attempting to sell. He entertains himself daily by enquiring about the soup, with no intention of ever purchasing any soup, just to watch the brief second of chaos as the staff try to figure out what is in the mysterious steaming vat on the back counter. It's usually minestrone, I've been reliably informed.

141 – Age-Appropriate Banter

Kids are cute and all, but let's be honest, I can outsmart most of them. Dr Upside-down, as I call myself when I peer down at them from the top of the bed so they're looking at me upside-down, has magical powers. Not only have I got the laughing gas, but I bet I can guess the name of your teddy or stuffed animal you've brought with you to theatre. Even more, I can smell your fingers and guess what you had for dinner last night.

It takes a while to get to grips with age-appropriate banter, and I'm still a long way from perfecting it, but it is an essential part of the job. I spend a lot of my day embarrassing myself in front of children. What I have learned, though, is that 90 per cent of the time I can guess the name of the stuffed animal. Some very close observation and years of dedicated focus has revealed to me that these super-imaginative little kids are in fact, quite unimaginative. A toy bear? That's 'Teddy'. A toy duck? That'd be 'Duck'. A toy horse? Oh, you best believe that's 'Horsey'.

Covert information-gathering occurs on the way to theatre. I stealthily apprehend Dad on the way down the corridor to procure information regarding last night's dinner. A quick whiff of little Billy's fingers and his head almost explodes in shock as I announce that I know he most certainly ate all the green beans with his chicken last night. After this, mesmerised, distracted Billy is only too happy to take the mask and start on the laughing gas.

I tried this tactic today on an older child, Jack, who has a moderate learning disability.

'Now I know you didn't have breakfast today but give me your fingers and I'll tell you what you had for dinner.'

'OK!'

(Whiff)

'Aha! Jack, you had spaghetti, didn't you?'

'Yes!'

'I knew it! You must be hungry if you haven't had anything since the spaghetti. We'll get you something to eat soon.'

'I had bread.'

'When did you have bread?'

'Over there,' he said, gesturing at the day unit.

'I see, did you now.'

A phone call later, and it emerged that Jack was seen exiting the pantry in the day unit where packets of sliced pan are stacked high for those returning from theatre. The door of the pantry, located very close to the post-op ward in the day unit, is almost always open. There is consistent traffic in and out as nurses and healthcare assistants cook up some golden, buttery toast to placate starving children after their operations. Jack, seeing his opportunity, probably just breezed in and helped himself. It wouldn't have taken James Bond levels of stealth. No one thought he had eaten anything, but a cursory examination of the room revealed the suspicious remains of at least two slices of white batch bread as the crusts were located behind the door. Surgery cancelled. Jack was delighted.

146 – Risky Business

Everyone expects to be faced with the death of a parent, but I hope I'm never put in a position where I'm faced with the mortality of my own child. It doesn't matter if you are told during pregnancy that your child has a fatal abnormality, or if you've known from a young age that they are unlikely to make it to their teens or even if they were healthy yesterday and some awful accident has them fighting for their life. No circumstance makes it easier to let a child go. Parents, by nature, are protectors of their children, their guardians. It goes against those evolutionary instincts to let a child pass away.

Most conversations about death occur in the intensive care unit. When treatment becomes futile, the medical staff must also become advocates for the kids and ensure any suffering is not prolonged. Almost everyone who is terminally ill in an intensive care unit will have an ETT, multiple cannulae, a urinary catheter, multiple monitoring lines and many more objects attached to their beds. Not to mention any pain they may have from the disease process itself. We do the best we can to ensure comfort, but it is not the same as being tucked up in your own bed at home.

Many parents know what is coming and only require medical staff to confirm their suspicions. They can accept that there is nothing more to be done. They have already begun to come to terms with it on some level. The difficult scenarios arise when there is a difference of opinion between parents and medics. Some parents will insist on pressing on with treatment that is already failing, despite medical advice to the contrary. We must tread cautiously by remaining objective and detached, but never without empathy. There is no easy way to convince a loving parent that their child is dying.

Today I was faced with a seriously risky anaesthetic for a child with a terminal cardiac condition. This stoic toddler had maxed out all treatment available and was on a slow and steady terminal decline. As the parents pushed for everything, advocating for their son, a relatively minor procedure was proposed as a possible measure to buy a bit more time. However, the process of being anaesthetised would almost certainly result in a further deterioration. No anaesthetist wants to have a patient have a cardiac arrest or die under their care, particularly for a non-life-saving procedure. This was a distinct possibility. I warned the parents that this risk of death was about 50 per cent. They accepted this risk.

They kissed him goodbye, wondering if it would be the last time that they saw him alive, and exited the department in floods of tears. Our surgeon worked as quickly as possible to try to minimise the time the child was under anaesthesia. The child's vital signs were shockingly bad, but this was his baseline. The goal was to keep this at the status quo and not push our luck. After 30 minutes we were done, and we started the process of waking him. He struggled to wake up fully, his oxygen levels even lower than when we started. I considered whether or not I should have just flat refused to anaesthetise him on the grounds of risk, but it is hard to say no to pleading parents. Another 30 minutes went by and he began to pick up a bit. The presence of his mum in the recovery room helped and his oxygen levels returned to their precarious baseline. We were, in all honesty, lucky. The parents were happy, but who was I treating here, the parents or the child? I went home considering if I did right by the child.

Postscript: he died two weeks later.

147 – Hugs

As I walk out of the radiology department, a child sits in a wheelchair in front of his mother. He is contorting his body around, almost 180 degrees, eyes wide open looking at who's passing him by. As I get closer, it is obvious he has Trisomy 21 (Down's syndrome). He looks about eight years old. As I get closer still, he gestures for me to come over. His arms open wide expectantly. He wants a hug. His fingers start to wag, urging me to hurry up. I open my arms too and catch him in a warm embrace. He means business, squeezing me tightly. After five seconds wrapped around me, his mum smiles and says the doctor has to go. He lets go of me and raises his hand in the air, this time for high-fives. I stroll off with my heart melting at his innocence. I turn around as I walk around the corner to see him again, arms wide open, gesturing at a six-year-old girl to come in for a hug.

148 – Shut Up and Dance

'OK. I want everybody to … floss!'

Suddenly the nurses and radiation therapists around me are gyrating and thrusting in an uncoordinated communal seizure. I haven't a fucking clue what's going on. We're all standing in a radiation therapy room, surrounded by clinical equipment and radiotherapy masks. Where are these instructions coming from? Is this a team-building exercise? Am I threatening the team bond by *not* thrusting? The voice comes on again.

'You too! Everybody! EVERYONE. FLOSS.'

The 'floss' is a dance (is it a dance?) that seems to have appeared in the last 12 months and gone viral. It involves fixing your feet in position and sort of diagonally thrusting your hips from side to side through a gate made by your two arms. I just keep thinking of Mr Bean. I cringe and commence gyrating. I glance at the other staff, some of whom I've met for the first time five minutes ago, and wonder where the hidden camera is. Are they setting me up? Is Ashton Kutcher here somewhere? *Come out, Ashton, I know you're behind that mirror.*

'OK! Now dab!'

Everyone looks flummoxed. My time to shine. The dab is something that I don't understand either (kids these days, huh?). It looks something like Usain Bolt's signature lightning bolt move except that what you want to do with a dab is bury your forehead into the trailing arm. Obviously, this all makes perfect sense. I start dabbing. Bang, one way. Bang, back the other. Dab, dab, dab. *Oh yes, nurses, now you feel silly not knowing how to dab. Eat your heart out, Paul*

Pogba. I'm leading the charge and I'm getting into it. I hope the moonwalk is next. I've been practising.

We hear the patter of feet in the corridor. He runs in, delighted. 'You know the dab!' he squeals. He high fives me as he jumps up onto the bed, ready now to be anaesthetised. Aaron is seven years old and on day nine of a 30-day radiotherapy course to treat his brain tumour. Every day requires a general anaesthetic. He knows his way around the department, including where the control room is. This room houses the monitors through which he can control the cameras that are focused on the radiotherapy suite. His new routine is to peer through the cameras, and demand dance moves of increasing difficulty down the intercom at everyone preparing the room for his treatment. We have no choice but to down tools and floss. *Just shut up and dance, Karen.*

152 – A Different Kind of Toff

Everyone remembers the major 'first times' in their lives. The first time I kissed a girl (in the bushes up the road in 1995), the first alcoholic drink (a lukewarm can of Heineken in 2000), the first cap for my country (I used to be ok at hockey – 2000). Is it sad to say that I remember so many of my first experiences in medicine? I don't think I'd be alone in admitting that. Some of them I recall because I never want to relive them again, some because it was a huge weight off my shoulders, others because I satisfied myself that I was capable. I remember the first time I felt like I could be a good doctor, after a specific exam in obstetrics. The first time I had to explain a diagnosis to a patient, for atrial fibrillation. I remember the first time I intubated someone, the first time I failed to intubate someone. The first patient I admitted and managed by myself in intensive care. The first patient I resuscitated after a cardiac arrest. I remember the name of the first patient who died under my care in intensive care. I remember the name of the first child I anaesthetised for a heart transplant.

Today, on an otherwise quiet Sunday afternoon, I was presented with another name that I will never forget. As the only consultant anaesthetist in the hospital, we plodded our way through some straightforward fractures and a few other nondescript cases. At around midday, I glanced outside to see the sun still splitting the sky. Fantastic, I thought, expecting to be out of the hospital by 3 p.m. to catch some of the remaining rays. Then the phone rang.

'There's a six-hour-old baby, weighing less than 3 kg, who has a trachea-oesophageal fistula. It needs to be repaired today.'

A trachea-oesophageal fistula (TOF) is a rare neonatal surgical emergency and requires surgery as soon as is feasible.[38] There might only be 15 in the country each year. It is an extremely challenging operation for the anaesthetist, and due to its rarity it's hard for any anaesthetist to become an expert in managing TOF cases.

I must admit, it is the one diagnosis I still had apprehension about managing by myself. I have never anaesthetised a baby for a TOF repair as a consultant and have only experienced one as a registrar. I feel a sense of focus wash over me. I call a senior colleague for advice and am most grateful when he answers the phone while playing with his kids in the sunshine. I am confident of what I am doing, but want reassurance that my plan is suitable.

---

38 As the name suggests (or doesn't suggest anything at all if you're not medically trained) there is a connection (fistula) between the trachea (windpipe) and the oesophagus (food pipe). It is most often accompanied by an oesophagus that is atretic – meaning there is no continuation between the upper and lower parts of the oesophagus. The atretic oesophagus means that the baby cannot swallow saliva and instead it pools in the back of the throat and can subsequently pour into the lungs. Or worse, gastric acid can spill up from the stomach, through the fistula and into the lungs. This all means that if it is not picked up quickly the baby's lungs can get severely injured very rapidly. We sometimes use the acronym TOF as shorthand for 'Tetralogy of Fallot', which is a disease of the heart. It can be confusing. Sometimes we call a trachea-oesophageal fistula a 'surgical TOF' and Tetralogy of Fallot a 'cardiac TOF', or a 'Tet' or a 'Fallots'. Very clear altogether.

Then I'm ready to get cracking. This is a big 'first' to get out of the way. I know I'll remember it as it is probably the most challenging anaesthetic we deliver in paediatric practice. In the end, everything went surprisingly well.

I'm not sure what it is about 'firsts' that cause them to be etched on our memories forever. They are intensely emotional experiences. While personal 'firsts' are often tied to friendship or love, medical firsts are inevitably tied to fear and anxiety. Knowing that someone else's life lies in your hands is a significant weight to bear and the overriding emotion afterwards is always relief. I remember them so vividly.

Maybe that's why my senior colleagues appear so relaxed all the time: they have no more medical firsts to bear.

154 – Beautiful Nothing

There is little more satisfying in anaesthesia than watching the scalpel of a surgeon plunge into the skin of the patient and see nothing happen. Never is 'nothing' so perfect. The nothing I'm referring to is not what happens next in the surgery. No, after that initial incision I settle back behind the surgical drapes to write my notes. The notes are all the easier to write when I see nothing. No change in heart rate. No change in blood pressure. No hyperventilation. No flicker of movement from the patient. Beautiful nothing.

This sort of reaction (or lack of reaction) to having your skin cut open is usually only possible with regional anaesthesia. Regional anaesthesia is sometimes called a 'block' or a 'nerve block', and it is the very best form of pain relief. We have many analgesic drugs at our disposal, but to achieve the nothingness like I described above with opiates, you need to use high doses and expect the consequences (e.g. they'll stop breathing, they may become nauseous). With a good regional block, the patient will feel no pain at all, breathe beautifully and one would hardly notice from their vital signs that surgery was even taking place.

It is called 'regional' anaesthesia as opposed to 'general' anaesthesia as you only switch off the lights in a certain part of the body, instead of turning off the entire brain as in general anaesthesia. Think of a power cut in your neighbourhood despite the power station still running as normal. The idea is that we flood a specific part of the nervous system with local anaesthetic drugs that block all sensory and motor function of the nerves. This means that, in that specific targeted area, you will feel no pain and will (usually) not be able to move a muscle. For example, an injection of local anaesthesia in the axilla (armpit) will render you unable to feel or move your arm. Another more common example is that of an epidural injection often used in labour that will render the patient unable to feel anything below the belly button.

It is common in adults to have entire surgical procedures performed awake, under the effects of regional anaesthesia alone. I had one myself. It was strange watching (I asked to see) the surgeon, a friend of mine, opening the palm of my hand with a blade sharp enough to slice through bone without any sensation whatsoever. In kids, however, we usually combine regional anaesthesia with general anaesthesia as the prospect of an awake child having surgery is not desirable to even the most patient healthcare workers or parents.

I slid an epidural catheter into an infant who was having a bowel operation today. It glided into position as is often the case in skinny kids. The true test always comes as the surgeon picks up the knife. You usually have a gut feeling if the block will be successful or not. My registrar looked at me as the surgeon asked for the knife, vial of fentanyl in one hand, syringe in the other. I shook my head and sat down. He of no faith. The icy blade pushed into the child's abdomen, and nothing. Sameness. Mundane, boring, beautiful nothing. It's what every anaesthetist dreams of.

156 – Have You Seen This Dog?

After I explain to both child and parents the process of anaesthesia and what to expect out of their experience on the big day of surgery, I ask if they have questions. More often than not, parents will have a query or two that can be easily answered. It's rare that parents have a question that I struggle to answer. Regularly, though, the inquisitive nature of kids leads to some questions that are nearly impossible to answer, most of which aren't remotely related to anaesthesia. I assume that some questions are repeats of those either avoided by parents or unanswered to the level of satisfaction of a seven-year-old. The best questions come from five- to ten-year-olds. A smart child usually seizes the open mike opportunity I present to hit me, another unsuspecting adult, with some of the hard-hitting issues discussed in the primary school playground.

'Why is the sky blue?'

'I don't know.'

'Do you think Ironman lives in Dublin?'

'Probably in a mansion in Dalkey, yes.'

'My friend Amy doesn't like this hairband. Do you like this hairband?'

'Eh, yeah! Amy sounds like a complete bitch.'

OK maybe not, but you get the idea.

I got a toughie today:

'Is Max in this hospital?'

'I'm not sure. Is Max one of your friends?'

'No, he's our dog!'

I don't like where this is going. I glance at the parents, who glare deep into my soul with frosty eyes.

'I'm afraid we don't have dogs in this hospital.'

'He's been in the hospital for ages.'

'Your parents are lying to you, just like mine lied to me. Our dog, Patch, went to the farm and never came back. I suspect poor Max will be in the hospital forever. Never trust an adult, little one.'

As much as I wanted to tell the truth and expose the parents as unadulterated liars, I refrained. I was happy when Mum interjected and steered the conversation away from poor, clearly deceased and never-to-return Max.

The kids over ten start to get more serious. I like getting asked sensible questions by patients. If my life were in the hands of someone I had just met and in a field in which I had no experience, I too would ask some real thinkers. The best question I was asked was by a young teenage girl in London. She asked me, 'How are you going to make sure you don't kill me?'

To give this question some context, I was due to anaesthetise this girl for a heart transplant. Only two weeks prior, she had been due to have elective minor surgery in a different hospital. She was thought to be an otherwise healthy young teenager. Following a standard induction of anaesthesia, she had a cardiac arrest. She was effectively dead for 15 minutes while she was resuscitated but, obviously, the outcome was good. Due to the skills of those resuscitating her, she regained consciousness with no apparent neurological injury. The cause of this cardiac arrest was an undiagnosed cardiomyopathy (disease of the heart muscle). Her heart was on its last legs and she was referred for a heart transplant.

'How are you going to make sure you don't kill me?'

What a loaded question from a smart kid. If you were told that in order to live, you had to bungee-jump off the Golden Gate Bridge, but the last time you did it the cord snapped, you crashed face-first into the water and almost died, would you do it? The only reassurance you receive is the safety man telling you, 'You'll just have to trust me this time.' Imagine the terror. I would sit that safety man down and get him to tell me, step-by-step, exactly how he was planning to keep me safe. I would pepper that poor bastard with question after question. *What is the cord made of? Have you*

checked it for bungee-ness? How long have you done this? Have
you been drinking?

'You think I might kill you? What do you mean exactly?'

'Will I go to sleep the same way as the last time?'

'More or less, yes.'

'Will you use the same drug as the last time? They used a white one.'

'Yes, we will probably use that drug as well as some others.'

'Well, if the white one nearly killed me, why are you using it again?'

Good question. Do we have enough time to explain the pharma-
cokinetics and pharmacodynamics of propofol?

'We put many kids with your heart problem asleep every week, so you're in the right place.'

'So did the other hospital not know what they were doing?'

I need to speak to my solicitor.

'They did know what they were doing but they didn't know you had a heart problem.'

'So would they not use the white drug if they knew?'

'Probably not.'

'So why are you using it?'

Good question. 'Propofol is an intravenous anaesthetic drug with a chemical name of 2, 6 – di-isopropylphenol ...'

'I'm not going to give you very much and we'll be taking it very slowly.'

'Ok, so the other guys gave me too much?'

WHERE IS MY SOLICITOR?

'Well, they probably gave you the normal amount for a kid with a healthy heart.'

'But now you know I don't have a healthy heart so you're going to give me just a little bit?'

'Yes.'

'Ok, then.'

In the space of 30 seconds this young woman understood the complexities of anaesthetising someone with end-stage cardiomyopathy. In all honesty, I could not guarantee her that she would not have another cardiac arrest on induction of anaesthesia. But she didn't ask me to guarantee anything. I think she was able to gauge the subtext of what I was saying and chose not to ask that specific question. She was one of the brightest kids I've come across and I'm glad to say that she not only survived the operation, but was up and doing homework in her hospital bed less than a week post-transplant. Her questions were tough, but give me those clinical ones ahead of predicting the outcome of a Royal Rumble featuring Batman, the Hulk, Magneto and Spiderman any day.

159 – Size Isn't Everything

The gargantuan proportions of some children make it easy for me to forget that they are, in fact, still children. A man-mountain strolled into theatre today for a minor surgical procedure. He was well over 6 foot, weighed more than 100 kilos and had some reasonably accomplished facial hair for one so young. I assumed that one of the porters had donned a surgical gown for a bit of craic until his tiny mother shuffled in behind him. A teenage brick shithouse. If he was from a different part of Dublin there would be rugby schools clambering over each other to sign this guy up as their new second-row forward, destined for the Irish team. I peer up at him and introduce myself. His knuckle-crushing handshake tells me he could squash me like a fly. Our operating tables are not set up for someone of his proportions as his feet (along with half of his calf muscles) dangle off the end of the table.

'You must be a rugby player?'

'No.'

'Gaelic football?'

'No.'

'Football?'

'No.'

'Basketball then!'

'No.'

'Any sport?'

'Not really, I play *FIFA* on the Xbox.'

My hopes that the Irish soccer team would have a new towering, commanding centre-back in the coming years are dashed. A loss to Irish sports.

The first reminder that he is, as his date of birth suggests, a teenage boy is the cringe, squirm and yelp that he releases as I poke a tiny needle into the back of his hand. He looks at his mum for reassurance that everything will be ok. She strokes his hair and holds his other hand. *Mate, you're going to have to man up if you're going to keep Romelu Lukaku quiet. Oh wait, you're just a teenager.* I switch back into paediatric mode as I send him drifting off to sleep. But the doses I use resemble the 'one-vial' anaesthesia more accustomed to adult practice. Everything in paediatric practice is weight-based, including drug doses, so we spend a lot of time calculating doses to make sure we don't overdo it. However, in his case, I am comfortable emptying a full vial of propofol, fentanyl, atracurium and the rest. The endotracheal tube we have selected more closely resembles a garden hose than the tiny tubes we are used to. We have to go searching for a blood pressure cuff big enough to accommodate his bicep.

Post-op, I am once again reminded that he is still a teenager. He has some pain in recovery and I am asked to review him. The (relative) masses of fentanyl and morphine he has received would send most of our kids to intensive care to sleep it off over a few hours, but not him. He, unfortunately, is still sore. Mum again holds his hand as a few lonely tears roll down his cheeks. *Damn it.* Being pain free (or close to it) is one of the core jobs of an anaesthetist. Maybe his size threw me off; maybe if he were in an adult hospital

I'd be more comfortable giving large doses. A little bit of extra pain relief helps him significantly. He's now happy and chatting with us and has only one question:

'When can I go back to the gym?'

Wait here, I'll call Andy Farrell and tell him you're ready. There's still a chance you'll make the Six Nations.

160 – A Casual Day in Work

Consider this scenario: you wake up one morning, relaxed and ready to go about your day. You arrive in work and check your diary. There are just a few straightforward meetings in the morning, followed by a leisurely lunch. The afternoon brings a team-bonding exercise followed by a yoga class. All in all, it's looking like a great day. As you casually stroll to the meeting room, cupping your smooth flat white in one hand, laptop in the other, you hear a rumbling. Sounds like someone is running. Before you know it, you are rugby-tackled into the back of a Ford Transit. Frothy coffee flies through the air, you hear the laptop crack against the pavement. A bag is thrown callously over your head. In the back of the van, there is commotion. Voices shout profanities, unfamiliar sounds make strange clicks and beeps. You are laid flat on the ground onto what feels like a dusty rug. The van stops suddenly, you feel your-self being rolled, like a sausage, into the rug. Three hundred and sixty degrees, twice. The door swings open, a cold breeze filters through the tiny perforations in the bag on your head. Two or three men, you're not quite sure, drag you out of the van and hoist you up to an uncomfortable height. You hear running water below. *Is this happening?* Gravity pulls you down, over the bridge. It seems like an age before you reach the water with a dull splash. Icy water rushes in and consumes you. It's the last thing you remember.

Until, you come to your senses. You are dragged from the water onto a rocky shore. Freezing and shivering, the voices tell you it's all over. *How long was I in the water? A minute, two?* A full 20 minutes after hitting the shocking water, you have emerged, alive. The bag is removed from your head, some familiar faces greet you and hand you some lukewarm coffee. You are guided to a car which drives you back in the direction of the office. The car pulls to a gentle stop and the door opens of its own accord. Suddenly, your laptop is back in your hand and you are being ushered into the meeting which was delayed given your mysterious brief disappearance. With your soggy clothes weighing you down and your mind racing, you shuffle into the meeting room. Your backside makes an audible 'squelch' as you sit down. 'Ok, what's next on the agenda?'

Ok, ok, I'm probably being a bit dramatic, but that's what work felt like today. The list of emergency operations looked very civilised in the morning, all healthy children for minor enough surgery. It would be a good day. My phone suddenly started hopping. First the ENT surgical registrar, then the respiratory consultant, both frantically telling me there was a critically ill child, with an airway emergency, who needed to come to theatre immediately. The rugby tackle into the Ford Transit.

The phrase 'airway emergency' immediately gets the attention of any anaesthetist. This usually means that someone has blocked their entire airway, or a portion of it, due to trauma, swelling, drug reactions, post-operative bleeding or inhaled objects. I probably don't need to spell it out, but this is not a good thing as it effectively blocks off the ability to breathe, either partially or completely. We can only manage for a matter of minutes with a blocked airway before we suffer a cardiac arrest, even less in a child. Anaesthetists, being airway experts, are tasked with securing a safe airway to maintain the ability to deliver oxygen to the lungs. But such is the variety and nature of airway emergencies that we often don't know what we're dealing with until we get started in theatre.

As I rush to the ward to cast an eye on the two-year-old boy that is in extremis, my mind starts to work on my anaesthetic plan. *How will I put him to sleep? What equipment do I need? What is the back-up plan?* I probably only have five minutes to get this right in my head. The child is not well. He has inhaled a peanut and following a period of stability he has rapidly deteriorated on the ward. His oxygen saturations are 83 per cent (normal is 97–100 per cent). He is panicking. He won't keep the oxygen mask on his face. His parents, naturally, are terrified. I call the operating theatre and tell them what I need to have ready before we all gently and slowly start the journey along the corridor and up the lift to theatre.

The most senior ENT surgeon is waiting for me in theatre, ready to go. I am delighted to see him; this won't be easy. We manage to send the child off to sleep, but the real fun hasn't started yet. We are being rolled into the rug, the door of the van is open. The plan will be for me to keep the kid breathing by himself, to anaesthetise his airway with local anaesthetic solution and then allow the ENT surgeon to pass a rigid bronchoscope into the throat, trachea and beyond into the lungs. A rigid bronchoscope, for want of a better description, is a long, hollow piece of steel with a light source and camera and through which the surgeon can pass various instruments. The saturations are up to 90 per cent with the supplemental oxygen.

Beyond the trachea, each lung is supplied with inspired air via a main bronchus, the left main bronchus to the left lung and the right main bronchus to the right lung. Our surgeon passes the bronchoscope for the first time and we see the problem: the peanut completely blocking the left main bronchus. A grasping instrument is passed into the bronchoscope and gently the peanut is snagged and removed. An audible sigh of relief reverberates around the room. Job done. He has another look with the scope, just to be sure, and then we see it, another peanut completely blocking the bronchus. We've been thrown over the bridge into the water.

The saturations are now intermittently dropping to 75 per cent when the bronchoscope is in, before recovering when it is removed.

There is a very short window to work in. We go again. Skilfully and slowly, the second peanut is removed. Another sigh of relief. The saturations come up again. One more look down to check, and guess what? Another peanut, again blocking the main bronchus. There is now some trauma and swelling in the airway due to the presence of both the peanuts and the cold steel instruments. I summon some help from a senior colleague. We now have two consultant anaesthetists, two consultant ENT surgeons, two anaesthetic registrars, two ENT registrars and about eight nursing staff. All for a few peanuts.

The third peanut is hard to retrieve. It is deep in the left main bronchus and the child coughs when the bronchoscope tickles the airway this far down. The local anaesthesia is hard to disperse to this depth. Not a good combination. But he is resilient, and we are managing – just. It will take one last mammoth effort to get this third peanut out. Everything is poised, a deep breath in from everyone. In goes the bronchoscope. We contort the child's body into a position to give the best view of the offending nut. By turning the head to the right, we get better straight alignment between his mouth and the left main bronchus – the bronchoscope being rigid and completely straight. The forceps are out again. The peanut moves and bobs, ducking like a champion boxer's head. A nip and gentle tug and our surgeon has caught the little bugger. Out comes number three before another glance inside. A fourth peanut. However, this one is not blocking the bronchus so we can now get some precious oxygen into the left lung. The saturations come up to near normal levels. Our heads are above the water.

The last peanut is easy to retrieve but we know he will have significant trauma, swelling and probably a nasty infection in the lungs in the coming days. As we discussed with the parents, we elect to send him, minus his peanuts, to intensive care. We are being pulled out of the water. I drop him back to intensive care and explain everything to his extremely relieved and grateful parents.

I walk back to theatre, already mentally exhausted, and it's not yet 9.30 a.m. The next patient is already there. Dry yourself off and get into the meeting, a full day or work awaits, no time for a glass of water. I love it.

162 – Tee Time

According to one of my nursing colleagues, I've already become a caricature of a consultant. A bit harsh, as all I did was enquire if she's seen any of the golf over the weekend. A major tournament had been all over the TV. I probably should have started the conversation with something other than, 'Do you play golf?' I mean, I don't actually *play* golf. I hack my way around a golf course once a year. I can appreciate talented sportspeople is the thing. The reply was damning.

'Oh, for fuck's sake, Colin, the state of you! You're a real consultant now.'

'But … but …'

'No, I don't play golf! What tournament are you even talking about? You'll be telling us about your five-star resort holidays next. Or your new Mercedes. Cop on to yourself.'

It was all tongue-in-cheek, but I can see how consultants don't do themselves any favours in trying to alter public opinion of themselves (if indeed they do talk exclusively about golf, fancy holidays and flashy cars). Would the response have been the same if I had asked if anyone saw the hurling at the weekend?[39] I laughed it off and the whole notion of the stereotypical consultant, safe in the knowledge that us *new* consultants are *different*. Approachable, grounded and relatable. I sat with a surgical consultant at lunch.

---

39 For the record, I am not a member of a golf club, our next holiday is in Cork and I don't even own a car.

'Have you been watching the golf? I'm staying in Adare Manor next weekend, should get a couple of rounds in. And hopefully a holiday in California to play Pebble Beach soon.'

166 – Mobile Pharmacies

Apparently, the most common drug error we make as paediatric anaesthetists is with paracetamol. That's right, plain old paracetamol that you pick up in the pharmacy and lob down your gob like Smarties to cure almost all that ails you. It works for kids too, of course. That delicious sugary, syrupy Calpol almost tasted like a treat for me as a child. Headache? Calpol. Growing pains? Calpol. Crying at night? Calpol. Annoying Dad while he's driving? Calpol. *I'm trying to watch the football! Where's the bloody Calpol?!*

Dosing almost all drugs in adults is relatively simple as there is usually a one-size-fits-all recommended adult dose. Therefore, administering drugs for anaesthesia in adults can sometimes be as easy as 'one vial of that, one vial of this and one vial of that over there'. Not so easy in children as all our drug-dosing is done in millilitres/milligrams/micrograms per kilo of body weight. A large chunk of our day is spent doing mental arithmetic or for those not so sharp on the numbers front (myself included) using a calculator to make sure we deliver the correct dose. Minor overdosing or underdosing is usually of no clinical significance. However, major overdosing can have significant adverse effects and thus we are anal about drawing up and checking drug dosages. No other medical specialty draws up and administers medication as frequently as anaesthetists. We are like mobile pharmacies.

I found it surprising then, as you might too, that a common drug like paracetamol is the source of most of our errors. One major factor is that we give it to almost everyone. Therefore, proportionally it accounts for most of our errors, but the error rate of administering paracetamol is probably very low. Much like we see more trauma caused by car crashes compared to trauma from those who fall from a window. But the vast majority of car journeys occur without incident, whereas everyone who falls out a window gets hurt. Driving is still safer than jumping out of fifth-floor windows. Paracetamol is still a very safe drug.

We had a case of 'too many cooks' today as I was assigned two registrars. Inevitably, we had a drug error. Almost two in fact. The three of us anaesthetised a child who was effectively adult-sized (a young teenager over 75 kg) for a major operation. Strangely, the error occurred in the opposite manner to which you'd expect. Before every major surgery we administer antibiotics before the surgeon puts knife to skin. I managed to spot registrar number two about to give antibiotics despite registrar one having done so only moments before. I gave myself a big pat on the back, and we all had a great conversation about human error, human factors and the importance of communication. Well done us. Until a bit later on, when they both gave the patient a dose of intravenous paracetamol without checking with the other. *<facepalm>* Double-dosing paracetamol once like this in a person this size will have no adverse effect. It would potentially be worse in a small baby, though.

This brings us on to a favourite topic in medical ethics: open disclosure. While it is very clear that if a serious adverse event occurs anywhere in medicine, then it is our duty to disclose what happened. In addition, the patient has a right to know everything about their medical care. Yes, it is a bitter pill to swallow, and occasionally embarrassing, to admit when you have made an error. But it is well described that the outcome and resolution of any conflict resulting from medical error is better served by those involved being forthcoming and accountable for their errors. Anaesthesia is a very interesting specialty in this regard as, if you are doing your job correctly, the patient will not be aware of any error having occurred. You might even be thinking that we could 'get away with it'. But that, of course, is unethical.

The ethical guidance is less clear for errors that didn't actually result in any harm. If your car bumper gently came into contact with the bumper of the car behind you while parallel parking, would you wait around to explain that there is no damage to the other person's car? Not infrequently, events occur under anaesthesia that would not be normal on a general ward. For instance, if a patient on a ward has pneumonia and they are left with low oxygen levels, and nobody gave them oxygen, then this is an adverse event. If a patient's oxygen saturations briefly dropped during induction of anaesthesia, is it an adverse event? I would say not, as this is within the expected range of clinical anaesthesia. We would otherwise spend most of our day apologising for the fleeting abnormalities in vital signs.

We discussed our double dose of paracetamol and decided that, although it was not of any clinical significance, we would tell the patient and parents, neither of whom cared and looked at us as if we were making a mountain out of a molehill.

170 – Breaking Bad

I am glad that I don't work in a specialty that has to break bad news to patients of families very often. In fact, if you work exclusively in anaesthesia, you will likely never have to do such a thing. There may be the occasional minor morbidity (like some post-operative nausea or vomiting) from anaesthesia, but a death or major adverse event is exceedingly rare. I greatly admire those who do have those difficult conversations frequently. I see it in my wife after she comes home from a busy day in a urology clinic having told five patients that they have cancer that day. It's hard not to become emotionally involved, but also important to remain somewhat distant, otherwise the job would be unsustainable.

I had a rare experience today: it was me who broke some bad news, albeit not with any words, but more with what I didn't say, and the expression on my face. Yesterday, I anaesthetised a toddler who had been unwell for about two weeks with shortness of breath before his mother brought him to the ED a couple of days ago. He was found to have fluid around his vital organs, which indicates that something is seriously wrong. He came to theatre to have a drain inserted to remove the fluid from around his heart, the volume of which was so large it was impairing the ability of the heart to function.

Interested to see how he was recovering, I went to visit him and his mother this afternoon. The nurses informed me that 1.5 litres of fluid had drained from inside this very little boy. He looked brighter, but you could easily tell he was unwell. The swelling from the fluid was still present, giving the impression he was a lot chubbier than he truly was. As I chatted to his mother, she asked me about the results of the blood samples he'd had, the CT scan and what they had found in the fluid we had drained. I said I didn't know, which was the truth. She told me an entire team of doctors had arrived that morning, but no one had told her exactly what was happening.

'I think it's cancer,' she said to me. I pursed my lips and looked back at her. She started crying. I thought about my words and chose them carefully. I was out of my area of expertise, but it was almost definitely a cancer of some description. I allowed her to explain why she thought this was the case. After coming to her own conclusions, the best I could do, and probably the most I should have done in the circumstances, was agree that cancer was high on the list of possible diagnoses.

Much like the rushed outpatient clinics where bad news is broken every day, I had no more time to spare for her, as my next patient was waiting in theatre for me.

171 – Dead Mexicans

When you become a paediatric anaesthetist and you fully commit to a lifetime of working with kids, it is desirable, nay, *essential*, to purchase some colourful and thematic scrub caps. The alternative is the single-use, paper-thin, unstylish and probably environmentally unfriendly one-size-fits-all blue caps you find in all hospitals. How boring! How else am I supposed to express myself? How is anyone supposed to know you support Arsenal? Or like Harry Potter? How do you hint that you might have a bit of substance to your personality outside the hospital?

When I moved to London for my fellowship, this signalled to me that I was in this paediatric business for the long haul and I pressed the order button on my first set of scrub caps. Meaning to buy three caps, I bought seven, including the snowman Xmas one I can only wear for one week per year. *This is it, there's no turning back now, you've spent $35 plus shipping for these bad boys. Paediatric anaesthesia it is.* Great Ormond Street Hospital had some expressive individuals. Some had a scrub cap (and matching lanyard) for every house in Hogwarts. Some made their own *Game of Thrones* hats as they couldn't find any online. My first order was fairly tame, mostly science themed with a hint of cats and some Mexican skulls. In hindsight, selecting a scrub cap with Mexican 'Day of the Dead' skulls for work in a children's hospital may have been ill-advised. But the Mexican kids all love them, so why not everyone else?[40] It's all about the little victories in life. I don't know what I expected with my colourful hats. Maybe I thought the kids would love them, clap and smile as they picked out the chemical structure of actinine from my cap. *Hooray for Dr Science!* Alas, this never materialised. Dejected, there were times when I thought, 'What's the point?' Shall I bury them in my locker and simply conform with a standard-issue blue cap?

---

40 Note, I have not anaesthetised a Mexican child.

As I donned my Mexican skull hat and headed up to theatre, I expected more of the same – complete and utter ignorance of my amazing hat from swathes of foolish children. The day began just as expected until a dour-looking infant Adam appeared in the anaesthetic room. He looked to be on the border between laughing and crying, not a good start. I talked to his mum as she sat in a chair with Adam on her lap. I kneeled to the floor to show him the mask I would use to anaesthetise him. He looked up and gave a brief smile. I dropped the mask on the floor and bowed my head to pick it up. Suddenly, the heavenly laughter of an infant filled the room! *What the …?* I looked at him and he smiled. I bowed my head and he giggled. *Is this it? Is it the hat?* A look. A smile. A bow. A laugh. A look. A smile. A bow. A laugh. Today was the day – he was laughing at my scrub cap.

After what was probably close to ten minutes of me indulging my ego, we felt we should probably press on with the anaesthesia and surgery. His giggling mum agreed as I told her this had never happened before. This post is dedicated to Adam, the freaky little weirdo who made my day.

177 – Pancakes for Breakfast!

Three of our five patients today did not follow the simplest of instructions. Actually, I'll correct that: their parents did not follow the instructions. Maybe I'm expecting too much, but really, how hard is it? When a parent receives the call about when their child has been scheduled for surgery, they are given three nuggets of information:

What day to turn up
What time to turn up
When to stop feeding your child

So far, I think you'd all recognise my amazement at some people's inability to show up on the right day and time for what I would have thought is a major event in a young child's life. Now I turn my amazement to the complex world of fasting times. Except that it's not complex at all, it's quite simple.

Our fasting times before surgery are as follows – six hours for solid food, four hours for breast milk (not cow's milk or formula) and one hour for clear fluids. If you have a breastfeeding baby due to turn up at 8 a.m., you will be told not to give the child any breast milk after 4 a.m. If you have a teenager coming for surgery, you will be told not to provide them with any breakfast. The instructions are very clear. I thought.

I'm sure you can tell I'm writing out of frustration on this matter. I completely acknowledge that some information can be missed when parents are stressed about a hospital visit or dealing with other issues at home. Even getting a kid into hospital can be tough on some families in difficult circumstances, but it is important to the anaesthetist to know what's in (or preferably not in) the tummy of little Sophie. I'll have you all know there is a legitimate reason for all this faff. When you are anaesthetised, all your muscles become more lax and supple than when awake. This includes your gastro-oesophageal sphincter, which is what keeps your food from regurgitating back up your throat and continues its journey into the small bowel when ready. Needless to say, it is unwise to have a belly full of food when this sphincter relaxes under anaesthesia and the acidic contents of the stomach start to slide back up towards the throat. The acidic contents of the stomach are designed to digest food, not digest your lung tissue. Aspirate that muck into the lungs and you will be facing a spell in the intensive care unit.

We do not insist on these fasting times for the craic, just to terrorise your child who is already cranky at the prospect of a trip to the hospital. It's actually to ensure their safety under anaesthesia.

I can empathise with the fact that a hungry baby can be so distressed that their piercing cry is like an ice pick to the frontal lobe of an exhausted parent. But we attempt to minimise these fasting times as much as possible by providing some sugary clear fluid up to an hour before surgery, for example. A poor substitute for a delicious, mashed parsnip or whatever else your portable poo-factory is into these days, but it's the best we can do.

Today's list went as follows: Child 1 did not turn up and parents were not contactable. Good start for a surgical list that has a nine-month waiting list. Child 2 arrived at 8 a.m. with a belly full of her 6 a.m. breakfast that her mother chose to give her as she was cranky, meaning we could not anaesthetise her until midday. Child 3 arrived early, followed all instructions and was whisked as soon as possible into theatre to get things moving. Child 4 arrived at 10.30 a.m., on time, with a belly full of a significant portion of his father's petrol station breakfast roll consumed on the way to the hospital. This ensured that he could not be anaesthetised until about 3.00 p.m.

An idle operating theatre is a huge waste of hospital money (paid for by you, the taxpayer), time and resources. Personally, I don't mind staying late in work as many kids have travelled from the other side of the country or there are extreme social circumstances that mean cancelling their operation is not in their best interests. Not infrequently we operate on children who are cared for by social services, or by elderly grandparents, and even the process of obtaining consent can be troublesome. In those tricky scenarios, where it's hard to get all the ducks in a row on a given day, it's best to stay late and get the job done.

Overrunning theatres also have knock-on effects for the on-call team who may have to wait until well after 6 p.m. to commence any emergency surgery that is waiting in the wings. It seems every minute we lose at the start of the day adds on two at the end. But I'm not sure how we can be more explicit with our instructions to parents on preparing their child for the big day out in the hospital.

178 – A Fine Balance

I seem to be forgetting that working with children is all very new for most of our trainees. Some seem terrified of making an error and thus tread with inhibiting caution. But they can be overcautious to the point where I am being asked about every single minor decision. What size cannula to put in, what dose of paracetamol to give, what temperature the room should be, what colour socks they should wear. If I have stepped out of the room briefly, simple tasks may not be carried out until I return, for fear of retribution. There can be a distinct lack of initiative and thus I have found myself having to be very explicit with my instructions for each case to ensure that we all feel comfortable with the plan.

Being honest, I shouldn't really feel aggrieved if the junior staff are cautious in their approach to managing children. I, too, am cautious. But it does become tiresome when we are performing the identical procedure five times in a row and each time I get asked the same questions about how we will manage the next one. *Actually, this time I was thinking we might go old school and just hold him down and stick a wooden spoon between his teeth to bite down on for the pain. Or maybe a baseball bat to the back of the head? That should knock him out! What do you think?*

I'm being facetious. I was once a complete novice at this too. I used to hate consultants who would scowl at my inability to perform a simple task, even if the task was new to me while they performed it expertly every day of the week. I'm finding it a bit difficult to hit the communication sweet spot with some of the trainees. On the one hand, the group that are asking me the same questions repeatedly seem to want to be told *exactly* what to do during each case and so I've started spelling it out. But the level of basic detail I am spelling out is so elementary that if I was receiving it I'd think the person delivering it was an insufferable control freak and my eyes would be (figuratively) rolling to heaven. On the other hand, I'm learning to gauge those trainees who just get it straight away and with whom this approach would be detrimental to their independence and my patience.

The whole point of training is learning to become independent. As I trainee myself, if the consultant was not around, I would use my better judgement and make a decision myself. In medicine, if you can justify your decisions with evidence then you can soldier on comfortably. If you are practising with guesswork, then best you check yourself and seek clarification from a senior. Anaesthesia in particular is all pattern recognition: if you can't see the pattern through the waves of data points hitting you during an operation, then you're not ready to make key decisions just yet. This is all well and good if a trainee recognises their limitations. The problem of being a consultant, I'm learning, is when an overconfident trainee thinks that they see a pattern that doesn't exist and misses the real pattern.

So, I relinquish some control to trainees and supervise from a distance. Some need to be guided with baby steps and others need to be let loose, but with a critical and observant eye.

184 – Michael Jackson

More tricky questions from well-read teenagers today. Who's been giving them all these books? What's wrong with the PlayStation? *Hasn't anyone shown you how to spell BOOBIES on a calculator yet?*

We're ready in theatre to induce anaesthesia after placing a cannula in the back of Patrick's hand. I lift up a syringe of propofol – the white one, and by far the most common intravenous method of inducing anaesthesia.

'I know what that is.'

'Oh, you do, do you?' I was expecting some childish nonsense about it being milk, if I'm honest.

'That's propofol. That's the drug that killed Michael Jackson.'

You're not wrong, Patrick. I ponder if this is going to be an issue as Patrick, delighted with himself, swings his head over to meet the gaze of his mother. She doesn't smile as heartily as he does, more of a small nod of acknowledgement and the forced smile you give to a partial stranger when you pass them in the corridor. Patrick continues.

'Yes, his doctor gave him too much of it, and he died. His doctor went to jail.'

Listen. Patrick. I know what I'm doing. That guy was a cardiologist, he didn't know what he was doing! He was treating him for insomnia. It was entirely irresponsible of him to use a dangerous anaesthetic drug, in a private home, with no experience in airway management and no appropriate equipment. Yes, you could argue he was forced into it by Michael, seeing as he was on a large retainer, but it doesn't excuse his actions. Some even posit that Michael overdosed himself, but that theory was rebuffed by renowned propofol expert Dr Steven Shafer using complicated pharmacokinetic modelling proving that intermittent boluses of small doses of propofol that Dr Murray claimed Michael gave himself were insufficient to achieve the blood concentration level found at autopsy. I safely administer this drug every day, Patrick, and if that's not good enough for you, well then I'll just have to ask you to leave.

'You're right, I believe he did, Patrick. Are you ok with me giving you propofol?'

'He was a heart doctor and you're not. So yes.'

No medical defence solicitors needed today.

190 – Diplomacy

You would think that having spent ten years training to be a consultant one would be ready for anything when you finally arrive in the hot seat. Unfortunately, our training is woefully inadequate in preparing us for the majority of what is expected of us. Before you fall off your seats, I'm not talking about the clinical work. We are well able to work within our areas of expertise. But it turns out, we should also be accomplished in management, human resources, accountancy, business development, mechanical engineering and political manoeuvring.

I have come to learn that this takes up a huge amount of our time – much of it an annoying distraction when you are in the middle of clinical work. It's not particularly helpful when I am in the process of anaesthetising a baby to have a head pop into the anaesthetic room and ask me if I got the email about the 'INSERT NON-URGENT THING' they sent me. *Please go away for a while. Can't you see I am looking after someone's baby?*

Doctors like to think they are well-rounded individuals. I think this is true for the most part. You can't expect to be a functioning member of a consultant body if you don't have some additional 'soft skills'. But it is a stretch to expect us to be familiar with the more developed skills such as writing business cases for additional equipment and services or organising departmental budgets. But perhaps the most challenging nuance to the job is being a political mediator.

Anaesthetists are considered generalists. We can, of course, provide anaesthesia, but we tend to know a little bit about everything. We know some cardiology. We know some nephrology. We know some general surgery. We are facilitators. We often act as the middlemen and ultimately are some of the key decision makers. This seems like a fantastic position to be in until you settle in and finally become accustomed to some of the internal politics. There are strained relationships between anaesthesia and surgeons. Between surgeons and other surgeons. Between nurses and consultants. Between anaesthetists and intensivists. Between medical teams and surgical teams. It is all there, bubbling under the surface. It is, after all, a work environment.

As we are the middlemen, we frequently get sent in to mediate in talks to resolve scenarios as tense as the Cuban Missile Crisis. We regularly meet Kim Jong-un in the DMZ to discuss dismantling his nuclear weapons. I, singlehandedly, convinced Donald Trump to delete his Twitter account. A colleague last week successfully negotiated the unconditional surrender of the real Osama bin Laden (he was living in a treehouse in the Midlands).

I feel I am still too fresh-faced here to be overly assertive with my opinion. My tactic is to let others talk amongst themselves and come to a resolution. If it is the resolution I was hoping for, then fantastic. I have avoided a squirmy conversation. If it is not the resolution I was banking on, then the time has come to try and put my little foot down softly, without harming anyone's toes, just to let them know that I have an opinion too.

I take my negotiating position from how I try to practise clinically, by being flexible. By being easygoing. That way, I reason, on the occasion when I do need something done urgently, then the new tone in my voice allows people to hear that I'm being serious, and they work faster to help me. If you're uptight all day long, then you're setting yourself up for a 'boy who cried wolf' situation. I try to facilitate as much as I can by doing everything I can to help my colleagues, surgeons or other teams. That way, when I do say no to something, that opinion is respected.

I love how I think this tactic works. *Awww that's cute, Colin.* That's why I'm still sitting in work, at 7.30 p.m., covering an additional operation that I generously and unselfishly facilitated as a form of political handshake. *Hhhmmm … maybe I'm a pushover?*

192 – Toaster Roulette

There exists a very strained relationship between hospitals and toasters. I don't know about you, but on the rare occasion when I burn a bit of toast at home, I just open a window and chuck another slice in. Not so in a hospital. When a slice of toast gets burnt in a hospital, it seems to reach a hellish level of incineration. Plumes of thick grey smoke spewing from the piping hot toaster pocket. *Looks like the cardinals need some more time.* After the thing cools down, a crumbling, dusty, shrivelled piece of a substance formerly known as 'bread' is plucked out. The halls stink of smoke, sometimes for days. Staff divert their tea breaks to other ends of the hospital to avoid confronting the stench. Why does this happen only in hospital? I have thought about this more than you would care to know.

It probably all stems back to the introduction of free sliced pan. A major win for the staff. No need to eat breakfast at home when you can grab a couple of slices in the tearoom before work. The problem lies in the fact that on any given day there are probably more than 100 people working in even a moderately large operating theatre. That's a lot of toasting action for the four-slice Argos discount toaster. Bread is loaded in on the minute, every minute. Like pints of Guinness after a match in Croke Park, stacked four-deep on the bar counter, ready to go. People grab what they think is their slice. Others forget about their slice entirely, distracted by their accompanying cup of tea. Inevitably, one poor little slice gets left in the toaster for two, three, four or even … five minutes. Cue the smoke.

I have worked in about ten hospitals over a ten-year window and there have been multiple 'major' toaster incidents. They are usually deemed 'major' by the hospital fire safety officer, who, for good reason, gets a bit hot under the collar whenever there is a whiff of smoke in the air. I worked in one hospital where toasters have been banned forever. We have had toasters confiscated for a day/week/

month under suspicious circumstances. Eating cold, stodgy sliced pan is not the same as that warm crispy goodness oozing in melted Kerrygold butter.

Our current toaster has served us well. Burning incidents are down 30 per cent since last year. We seem to have hit the sweet spot on the temperature setting. But recently, there have been troubling signs that all is not well. The dreaded half-toasted slice of pan, again today. Now if you only have a two-chamber toaster, it's easy to remember which filament is not working. But we have a large, six-chamber beast. *What the …? Only one side again? I wish I could remember which slot isn't working.* Toaster roulette. Like Robert De Niro in *The Deerhunter*, only with fewer bullets.

197 – Woe Is Me

I made an error today. The same error that a trainee made about six months ago. At the time I wondered to myself how that was possible. Turns out, rather easily. It wasn't a grave error. It didn't, in any way, influence or affect the safety of a patient or the care we provided. It was one of those 'I'm not angry, I'm just disappointed' moments. I felt angry at myself briefly. Then I rationalised my thoughts and realised that there are far worse errors that can be made. I sighed and sat, feeling sorry for myself, on a stool in the corner of the operating theatre like a scolded, bold child. Being one who enjoys ruminating (if you can't tell already), I sat and mulled it over. What did I do (or not do) that enabled me to do such a thing? I wanted to make sure I didn't do it again.

Firstly, I was working too fast. *Quick, quick, quick. Do this, do that, do the other. A fast anaesthetist is a good anaesthetist.* This, I decided, is the unsubstantiated perception of the new consultant: 'Others will be happy if I work quickly.' Yes, well they might, but there are tens of other factors that influence whether we finish work on time. I am only one of them.

Secondly, I felt pressured. I had chosen, on this occasion, to induce anaesthesia in the operating theatre (which we often do for minor, quick operations). The operating theatre is like a watering hole in the savannah – you can see all sorts of creatures wandering in and out, thirsty for work. We use anaesthetic rooms for that reason – to keep a room to ourselves in which to work.[41] Every door to the anaesthetic room has a sign saying something along the lines of, 'No entry, anaesthesia in progress.' Naturally, this sign might as well be on the back of the toilet door as it is constantly ignored. The primary culprits are surgical consultants who frequently burst in 'just to see the notes', when in reality it seems like they are there to give you the sense that they are ready and waiting for you. A gentle squeeze. Their presence in the anaesthetic room is not helpful and more senior colleagues will literally push surgeons out of the room.

A consultant anaesthetist I worked with previously would produce a wooden spoon from her bag every morning. Unfortunately, not to smack the surgeons on the bottom on entry, that would have been way better, but to wedge in the door handles to effectively lock the anaesthetic room from the inside to prevent unwelcome visitors. Another colleague takes the phone of the anaesthetic room (which serves as the theatre phone) off the hook to avoid distractions. The important lesson from this is to work smart, not fast. Working smart means being more efficient with the time, maybe delegating a bit more and asking for help if you feel under some time constraints or are struggling with a procedure.

The other thing I mulled over, which actually bothered me more, was looking foolish in front of the trainee I was with. As a trainee myself, I have seen numerous consultants make errors and I could

---

41 Anaesthetic rooms usually adjoin an operating theatre. If you have a capable trainee, you can have one patient anaesthetised in the anaesthetic room, waiting for the preceding operation to finish in the theatre next door.

see the frustration in their eyes. Not once did I ever think they were foolish. If anything, it conveyed to me that consultants are not infallible. Medicine is hard and everyone is constantly learning. I hoped that by witnessing errors from seniors it would prepare me for becoming a consultant. For the most part, it has. But I can't hide from the fact that I felt like a fraud in front of the trainee. In reality, I doubt the trainee really cared that much and they learned the same lesson that I did over the years of training – nobody is flawless, and you can't get complacent in medicine.

198 – Speechless

I had an extremely high-risk infant, Saoirse, listed for a minor procedure today. Saoirse's condition meant she was too high a risk for a general anaesthetic, especially where there were other options to successfully complete the procedure. As I explained, first, why I felt the risk was too high, and, second, my alternative plan, her parents nodded in understanding and agreement. They asked sensible questions, understood my rationale and endorsed the plan in full.

I gave myself a small pat on the back. *Well done, Colin, you really are great at having these conversations. It looks like the family trust you with their loved one and we'll all be skipping and laughing together in a meadow soon.* As I was taught in medical school, I always end the conversations with, 'That's a lot of information to take in. Have you any more questions for me?' As Saoirse's mother shook her head, I had one hand on the door to leave. Unexpectedly, her father, who had just a moment ago been nodding in agreement, shot a sideways glance at his wife and hit me with a sucker punch: 'I'm not sure I trust you.'

After I assisted the accompanying nurse with retrieving her jaw off the floor, I let go of the door handle. *Well, that was surprising.* I don't actually remember what I said in reply: I may have giggled, I may have made incomprehensible noises, I may have winced as if my testicles were in a vice. My mind raced, wondering if my explanation was shoddy, if I seemed like it was my first day as an anaesthetist, if I had somehow suggested that my intention was *in fact* to fuck it all up for the craic.

'I'm sorry, I thought you were in agreement with the plan, Mr Davis?'

'I am. I mean, I think I am. But you've painted a bleak picture. I want to make sure she has the best anaesthetist, someone who's done this before.'

I could do no more than to repeat my plan, reiterating the fact that I had discussed this plan with senior colleagues, and reassure him that I have in fact done this before and that I am suitably qualified to do the job this time around.

Saoirse did not die, nor did she even so much as hiccup. In fact, everything went perfectly fine. But it took another 20 minutes of deep conversation with her father in her room before he was willing to allow me to provide the necessary care for his child. Parents or patients are perfectly entitled to ask for another opinion, or another doctor if they so wish. It makes me wonder how many more unasked questions there are in a hospital on a given day. Probably hundreds. Saoirse's parents didn't thank me in the recovery room. I'll get over it, and so will my ego. This isn't about me.

200 – Pride

I'm so very proud of him. I saw him when he arrived a few months ago. He was shy and quiet. He spoke only when spoken to. He was polite but needed significant direction in every regard. He was terrified of making an error. He made some clangers for sure, but they were usually minor, and it didn't take much to rectify them. He was attentive, though, and people were impressed with his technical ability. He worked quickly and professionally. His demeanour and attitude did let him down initially, though. The vacant stare as I gave my instructions did not fill me with confidence at times. I wondered if I should ask someone else to work with me instead. But, to be fair, over the last few months he has excelled. His work is phenomenal now. The way he looks at me, the way he just understands me. I have to say this is down to one thing only – a vast improvement in his communication.

When João from Brazil first started working in the café I didn't think he'd last long. His English was poor at best. But now he speaks with gusto and confidence and I'm even detecting a slight Dublin twang in the way he says, 'You having it here, or takeaway?' I look forward to our lunchtime chat. He knows what I want before I ask. We chat about the football and how he hates Neymar. *Me too, João*. I hope this relationship continues for many more years.

208 – Miracles

'Charge the paddles!'

The baby was in ventricular fibrillation. This is an arrhythmia that is not compatible with life. Instead of the heart muscle contracting in unison, different parts of muscle were contracting at different times, meaning the ventricles were wriggling, not pumping powerfully as they should be. No blood was leaving the heart. He was in cardiac arrest.

Now in ordinary circumstances this is a dire emergency that requires immediate use of a defibrillator to save the patient's life. But we were preparing to separate from cardiopulmonary bypass (CPB) after a long open-heart operation.[42] It is not uncom-

---

42 Cardiopulmonary bypass (CPB) is required to facilitate open heart surgery. When the main part of surgery is finished, with the heart stitched up again beating vigorously, we move to one of the riskiest parts of the operation. This is transitioning from the CPB machine doing all the hard work to the patient's heart taking over again. This is a gradual process, over a few minutes, and we call it 'separating' from CPB.

mon to see v.fib (as we call it) at this point of the operation. We were still on CPB, meaning that the baby was entirely safe. It can take time for the heart to return to normal sinus rhythm.[43] Nevertheless, we defibrillate the heart in these circumstances anyway as it is not healthy for the heart to be wriggling away in v.fib.

The surgeon grabbed the two long paddles used to defibrillate the heart, one in either hand, and gently straddled them across the heart inside the chest. After the instruction came to charge the paddles, we waited for the instruction to 'shock'. This would discharge the electrical current built up in the defibrillator through one paddle, through the heart and up the other paddle to complete the circuit. This usually restores sinus rhythm. We waited, but no 'shock' instruction was forthcoming from the surgeon.

'Aaaatchoooooooooo!'

Out of nowhere, our surgeon had let out a major sneeze. I glanced at the monitor. *Beep, beep, beep.* The electrically charged miracle sneeze had restored sinus rhythm.

218 – Guinness Farts

When an operating theatre is depicted on television it is often a quiet, tense environment where a stressed surgeon sweats to the relentless pulsating on the monitor. He (always a 'he') asks a nurse to dab his brow before there is suddenly chaos on the monitor before a cry of 'We're losing her!' shakes the cold, sterile room. This is an intense dramatisation of real-life events. Hospitals are more like *Scrubs* than *ER*.

---

43 Sinus rhythm is the normal heart rhythm. The initial electrical impulse for the heart to beat arises in the sino-atrial node, in the right atrium, causing the atria to beat in unison. The impulse travels through the atrio-ventricular node before spreading across the two ventricles, which then beat, milliseconds after the atria. It's remarkable.

Theatre is full of life and buzzing. Do we chat in theatre? Yes. The surgeons even chat to anaesthetists and nurses when operating. Do we listen to music in theatre? Yes. Unfortunately, the selection is usually at the discretion of the operating surgeon, meaning I have had to endure obsessions with ABBA, American country music and one surgeon who played AC/DC so loudly that we couldn't even hear each other speaking. Do we even have a bit of fun in theatre? Why yes, this can be known to happen too. It is, after all, our workplace and even we need to lighten the mood from time to time. There are stock stories in medical folklore. These include telling medical students that they must inform the surgeon if they have broken wind as otherwise the surgeon may confuse the odour with a potential perforation of the bowel. Or the surgeon who placed a false colostomy bag and an enormous dressing on the abdomen of an intern who was having a keyhole appendicectomy in the hospital in which he worked.

It was probably because I have not done today's list very often that I found the whole day quite hilarious. Much like everything else, unlike adults, a child will not tolerate an endoscopy or colonoscopy without a general anaesthetic. So here I was, providing just this very service. We wheeled the first child, a young boy, into recovery after his colonoscopy. As I handed the care over to the recovery nurse, someone in the vicinity let loose a fart so great it shook the curtains and woke the baby in the bay next door. It may have even melted part of the Arctic ice cap. I looked at the recovery nurse, horrified. Surely it wasn't her? She looked at me, smiled and motioned to the still unconscious kid.

'Do they all do this?!'

'Oh yeah, they all come out farting.'

In order for the gastroenterologists to have a good look in the stomach and bowel, the endoscope fills these cavities with air to expand them. They aspirate as much air as possible on the way back out, using suction attached to the scope itself, but it was quite evident that it's impossible to clear it all. Apparently, belching and flatulent kids fill Theatre 6 and the recovery area with a different kind of music several times a week. I sat there all afternoon entertained by the different sounds each rectum was making in turn. Some farts tried to escape as soon as the air went in, others sounded like someone teasing a tense balloon by marginally opening the orifice to let a high-pitched blast of air out. Most, though, sounded like any bedroom on a Saturday morning after far too many pints of Guinness the night before.

219 – Ward Rounds

Ward rounds are hilarious. Well, they're also mind-numbingly boring, but if you catch a good one it can be entertaining for a variety of reasons.[44]

Type 1 Ward Round: The Professor of Surgery

This type of ward round is characterised by a sartorially sound and enigmatic professor leading his exhausted team of registrars, SHOs and interns around the surgical ward. The crucial ingredient is the harem of medical students that follows the professor everywhere he goes. The group huddles around 'prof' at the bedside of Mrs Maguire, who has gallstones. 'Who can tell me the signs and symptoms of ascending cholangitis?' he asks expectantly. The medical students stare at their feet. One pretends to cough and goes to get a tissue. Another attempts to shuffle behind the tall surgical registrar. One attempts to divert attention by patting Mrs Maguire on the hand and asking how many cats she has. Another

---

44 One of my top three reasons for becoming an anaesthetist was that there are no ward rounds. Completing the top three were: not having to wear a tie and doing cool shit nobody else can do. However, we do partake in ICU ward rounds in our anaesthesia training, but these are only a fraction as dull as a general internal medicine ward round.

dives directly through the plate-glass window onto the bonnet of a Ford Focus in the car park below. Prof sighs and tells the most junior surgical trainee, Sarah the SHO, to tell the medical students the answer. Sarah looks at the registrar, who averts her gaze. You, the intern, grab a seat and get some popcorn for the show. *Sarah doesn't fucking know either! Prof is going to go through her for a shortcut!*

Type 2 Ward Round: The Post-call Round

'Post-call' means you've been 'on call' the night before. Consultants do not stay in the hospital on call, but registrars do 'in-house' call for most specialties. Actual restful sleep is not really an option; it's more of a fully clothed state of semi-consciousness with one eye on the pager. Those staying 'in-house' at night include general medical registrars but also anaesthetists covering intensive care. Sleep deprivation is apparently as disinhibiting as drinking alcohol. Don't believe me? Just watch a post-call ward round.

It's been 27 hours since I've got some sleep; why is this sadistic maniac asking me about potassium levels? I honestly don't care. What's next, an anecdote about when she went travelling in India? Yes, I'm sure it was difficult work, but do you know what else is difficult? Standing upright. Look at the man in bed nine there, in that comfy, automatic bed. He might have been in a car crash, but he doesn't know how lucky he is, all comfy over there on that soft mattress. He should try steering this car-crash of a ward round. Please let me just go home. Maybe if I just say, 'All the patients are grand' and walk off, I could get away with it. Shit, I haven't brushed my teeth for 28 hours and we're about to talk to that nurse I fancy. Maybe she won't notice. Oh no, I haven't been paying attention. Did she ask me something? Just nod in agreement – that should do. Maybe I should get a job in the United Nations; I'd say they do some good work. She's still looking at me – she definitely just asked me something. Just say '7.5' – that will cover urea, carbon dioxide, albumin, pH, haemoglobin, length of ICU admission, ET tube diameter and patient shoe size.

'The potassium is 7.5? Jesus Christ, someone get some insulin!'

Shit, I should've known it was potassium.

Type 3 Ward Round: Is There a Bed Available?

I slid up to PICU this morning for the same reason as many other consultants and registrars. To check the bed situation. For many major operations, we need to have a post-operative PICU bed and therefore cannot start surgery until we get the green light from the PICU consultant. Our intensive care is painfully over-subscribed and every day we gather outside the Sistine Chapel, waiting for the white smoke.

ICU rounds can be massive affairs at the best of times, with doctors, nurses, pharmacists, physiotherapists, nurse specialists, medical students, the Italia '90 team, Genghis Khan's army and leading figures from the 1916 Rising all trying to listen in to the discussion of the day's management plan. Early this morning I spotted a cardiac surgeon, three cardiac surgery registrars, three consultant anaesthetists, two cardiologists, a cardiology registrar and a general surgeon all slowly tip-toeing around at the back of the ward round, waiting for the correct moment to stake their claim to a bed. If they interrupt too soon, they may annoy the PICU consultant. If they interrupt too late, the available bed may be allocated to someone else before they even make their case. The bed is the North Pole and we have Russia, the United States and Canada with their flag poles in tow. I don't really get a say in the matter, but the poor PICU consultant has a tough job on her hands. You'd need a degree in international relations and experience in diplomacy with Fidel Castro before the discussion opens on who gets the single, precious intensive care bed.

A little core forms in the throng of the ward round with consultants from all specialties getting their brief audience with the PICU consultant. I'm in the second of the core circles, with an ear on the conversation. I'm eager to move as we have a long case ahead of us and each minute left discussing is a minute lost in theatre. Then the voices get raised a little. The discussion borders on argument. Eyebrows raise around the room. Who's going to win? It's looking like cardiology. They've played their hand well, classic manoeuvring. Russia has emerged victorious with a cheeky threat of all-out nuclear war. It's important not to use that one too often.

Without a PICU bed for our patient, I saunter back to theatre to see if I can be of use diffusing any more conflict.

220 – Persistence

'BOOOOOOOOOOM!'

What the fuck is going on?!

'I got it!'

This outburst was all the more surprising considering we had spent the last six hours in almost complete silence. No, nobody had dropped their wedding ring down the sink. Nope, we weren't searching for an elusive appendix (at six hours that would make it the longest appendicectomy since the Middle Ages). No, it wasn't the last clue in the crossword. It was our cardiologist expressing his sheer delight at finding the needle in the haystack.

Electrophysiology is a subspecialty within cardiology. It is the study of the electrical conducting system of the heart and for all intents and purposes it's pretty complicated. What is amazing is that the heart is a synchronous mass of muscle, with each muscle cell (myocyte) singing in unison to the same beat from the same hymn sheet. At least this is what occurs in a normally functioning heart. The metronome of the heart lies in the right atrium. From here, pulses of electrical activity travel through a specialist electrical conducting system to fan out to both sides of the heart. The result of this synchronicity[45] is the soothing 'lub-dub' sound of the heart-beat as the electrical conducting system means the atria contract first, followed milliseconds later by the ventricles.[46]

Unfortunately, like everything else in the body, things can go wrong on occasion. This system can be faulty for many reasons. The end result being a potential 'arrhythmia', or abnormal heart rhythm, some of which are lethal. Arrhythmias can be treated with medications, pacemakers or occasionally with an ablation procedure.[47] Ablation procedures are where electrophysiologists come into their own. Under anaesthesia, they insert long catheters into the veins in the groin and thread them up to the heart. From here the electrophysiologist uses very complicated-looking machines to make a map of the inside of the right atrium. I have tried my best to fully understand what they are looking at but fear I am still way off. The best I can do to describe it is to imagine a stockbroker (well, what I imagine a stockbroker does) looking at eight computer screens with continuous stock tickers, colours, lights, patterns, graphs and occasional alarms. The electrophysiology equipment is the medical equivalent of that.

From here the search begins for the microscopic pathway of cells that are causing the unwanted arrhythmias. To the untrained eye, this looks like the electrophysiologist wiggling tiny little wires repeatedly with no observable pattern before asking an assistant to turn on a pacemaker set to heart rates designed to murder the patient. That's what I see anyway. We sweat as our monitors scream at us to put an end to the madness. But as it continues into a second

45 I've always loved this word since The Police album of the same name and never thought I'd ever write it in a sentence, until now.

46 The sounds you hear when listening to the heartbeat is not the contractions of the muscles, but actually the valves within the heart snapping shut.

47 I spell 'arryhtmia' wrong every single time I write it. Arrhythmia? Arthmyia? Arhymthia?

hour, we become less worried about the heart rate of 200 beats per minute.[48] After a couple of hours, we're chatting to the nurses. After three hours we're lucky to be still awake. It is literally the medical equivalent of searching for a needle in a haystack.

You have to admire the persistence of the electrophysiologists. Long after I would have voluntarily electrocuted myself, they still search for the elusive pathway. The idea being that when they discover it, they obliterate the troublesome cells in the pathway from inside the heart (usually with heat) – this is the 'ablation' part of the procedure.

We had reached six hours today when the incessant seizures of our monitoring alarms had rendered me stupefied. The teenager had a condition that puts sufferers at risk of sudden life-threatening arrhythmias. They usually suffer no symptoms aside from very occasional palpitations. It is important to treat, though, to eliminate the risk of a fatal arrythmia occuring.

As is always the way with these sorts of things, our cardiologist turned to me and said, 'I think we're just about done here. I can't find the pathway,' dejectedly. Not two minutes later and I was holding onto my chair for dear life as the echo of the 'Booooooommmmm!' that burst from the gob of our electrophysiologist almost shattered the windows of the cath lab. He had found the pathway and was vivaciously letting us all know about it. He immediately ablated the cells. The ECG trace reverted back to what we would consider normal and all was well in the world again. Instantaneous gratification following monumental levels of persistence. Satisfaction.

---

48 The electrophysiologist isn't trying to kill the patient with these heart rates; he or she is trying to induce, or cause, the arrhythmia itself, to identify where exactly within the heart the abnormal conducting cells lie.

225 – Dr Butt, PhD

'Anaesthesia' and 'anaesthetist' are words that don't exactly roll off the tongue with ease. Maybe that's why some anaesthetists were upset that we decided to call ourselves 'anaesthesiologists' instead. I'm still stuck using 'anaesthetist'. There is something exclusive in being part of the minority of the population who can actually say 'anaesthetist' correctly. 'Anaesthesiologist' is slightly more straight-forward, but I can't help saying it in a markedly nasal American accent. It feels weird. *Hi, I'm Dr Black, anaesthesiologist.*

My own parents don't say 'anaesthesia' or 'anaesthetist' properly and I've long given up trying to correct them. The main issue is leaving out the sound of the first 's'. 'A-KNEE-thuh-tist.' 'Fraid not, it's 'a-NEECE-thuh-tist.' I have overheard other healthcare staff referring to us as 'the anaesthetic'. *Yes, the anaesthetic will be along shortly.* This is akin to saying, 'The cardiac will see you soon.' I'm definitely being pedantic, but the anaesthetist practises the medical role of providing anaesthesia to the patient using a series of anaesthesia-inducing drugs (anaesthetic drugs). I usually just introduce myself as the 'anaesthetic doctor'.

Today I met a wonderful girl who was extremely friendly and talkative. Children who share her diagnosis can suffer from some learning difficulties, but she certainly knew the ins and outs of her hospital visit. At first, she assumed I was the surgeon as I chatted to her and her mother about what to expect during her surgery. However, when I got deeper into the role I would be playing, the penny dropped for her. 'You're going to do my ass-thesis!' *Excuse me?* 'I had an ass-thesis the last time too.' Now, I don't have a PhD myself, nor have I ever had to write a thesis, but I'm pretty sure someone, somewhere has written a thesis based entirely on the ass. Be it the anatomy, function or just the things they love about a glorious rear end. As I fought back the tears of laughter, I had to just go along with it.

'Yes, I'll give you your anaesthetic today. How was the last one?'

'So, you're the ass-thesis?'

Ok so now I am the physical incarnation of the 10,000-word dissertation on the butt: 'Chapter 6: Hairy Arses'.

'Yes! I'm the anaesthetist.'

'Sometimes I get scared of the ass-thesis.'

I'm starting to get scared of the ass-thesis. *When is it due?*

226 – Backstreet Dentistry

Apparently, the thing anaesthetists get sued for most often is damage to teeth. I have heard stories of anaesthetists being sued after resuscitating patients from a cardiac arrest and accidentally damaging their teeth as they scrambled to insert a life-saving ETT into the lungs with CPR ongoing. *Sued? But ... but ... I helped to save your life ...*

Patients are often puzzled when we ask if they have any loose teeth or expensive dental work. We are not trying to steal your gold crowns when you are unconscious. When we send you off into the land of nod, we have to assist with your breathing or do it for you. This entails placing some sort of advanced airway device past your beautiful gnashers and into the back of your throat. The equipment we use can pass very close to your teeth or even touch them on occasion. Naturally, we don't want any rogue loose teeth falling into the back of your throat and into the trachea. Kids of all ages may have wobbly teeth, either 'baby' teeth falling out or sometimes rotting teeth falling out. So, there is reason for all the pestering about the state of your dentition. The official party line is that we don't want a loose tooth falling out and finding its way into your trachea, which is true. But really, we are trying to avoid litigation (well, I am anyway). More importantly, though, we don't want to scam a kid out of their tooth-fairy jackpot bonanza.

'Do you have any wobbly teeth?'

'Yes.'

'Will you show me?'

(Finger in mouth) 'Hrrrr, geerrre, heerre and hrrrr.'

Lizzy had four wobblers, two of which I just wanted to yank out. Being 99 per cent certain that they would fall out with only a gentle cough, I had to announce that I might have to catch them if they fell out when she was asleep. She (and parents) agreed this was ok and thus I carefully sidestepped any future dental litigation, this time anyway. Off she went to sleep and, sure enough, these teeth were hanging on by a thread so I grabbed a set of forceps and yanked the two of them out. We thought that *technically*, yes, she was asleep so therefore the tooth fairy would *probably* need to pay her for the teeth that came out.

One of the theatre nurses started a whip round. Fifty cent here, a euro there. Before long, she had almost €10 in the pot – a pretty decent return, I thought. The gravy train rolled over to the consultant surgeon, who announced that he didn't have any cash on him.

'Nonsense! I saw you stuffing a few €50 notes into your pocket in the changing rooms!'

He didn't laugh.

227 – What If

Thus far, most of my 'on-call' shifts have been very manageable. There have been days when we've worked up until midnight, but I have not had to put a child asleep after midnight. Yet. A full night's sleep in your own bed, whilst on call, is a dream come true and not a luxury ever afforded to anaesthetic registrars. I appreciate it all the more considering some of the exhausting night shifts we all went through as trainees. The sleeping quarters provided for registrars on call vastly differ in quality, ranging from a fairly plush en-suite room to cold and draughty Portacabins to nothing at all (thank you, NHS). The NHS feeling on the matter is that since you are rostered for a night shift, you should be working, therefore there is no need to provide you with somewhere to sleep. *But I put people to sleep for surgery ...? Am I to seek children for surgery? Shall I ring a bell on the street and advertise my anaesthesia services? Shall I mop the floors of the theatre?* When I arrive home as a consultant on call, I thank my lucky stars that it is into my own bed I am getting and not trying to build a little sleeping fort out of plastic pillows, under a table in some telecommunications storage room (NHS again).

But strangely, these remarkably calm on-call nights have not allowed me to settle nicely into life as a consultant. Quite the opposite actually. In the initial three or four months, I was excited to be on call. *What delights are going to arrive into the hospital tonight?* Finally having the responsibility to work entirely independently at night is a real test of your mettle. But as each quiet on-call has passed by with no real major challenge of my skills, a new anxiety is starting to build. Every Monday, the consultant who has just finished their weekend on-call usually vents or debriefs over coffee with some colleagues. They share tales of their difficult cases, how late into the night they were working, how the service was stretched or how they had to choose between two urgent cases at the same time. Recently, there have been some horrific Monday debriefs. A consultant who got less than five hours' sleep over their 48 hours on call. A consultant who had to rush a baby straight from the emergency department onto ECMO.[49] A consultant who had to push nearly nine bags of blood into a bleeding *baby*.

---

49 Extracorporeal membrane oxygenation (ECMO) is too complicated to explain in a note, but in a nutshell it is a method of preserving the flow of oxygenated blood around the body in cases of severe lung or heart failure or, more rarely, during a cardiac arrest. It is very similar, but not exactly the same, as cardio-pulmonary bypass. Venous blood is drained from the patient via an enormous cannula directly from the heart or a large blood vessel in the neck or groin. It is whizzed through a machine, outside the body ('extracorporeal'), that fills it with oxygen before whizzing it, via a centrifugal pump, back to the arterial side of the body via another enormous cannula.

Now, as my on-call day approaches my thoughts are consumed with the dread of the unknown. I have determined I am due something terrible. Some case so bad it will go down in the annals of medicine as the most complicated and horrific anaesthetic ever attempted. Has anyone ever had to resuscitate a baby during an earthquake in Dublin? *It's going to be me.* Has anyone ever had to deal with a bus carrying 30 children crashing into the very PICU some of them would need? *How ironic! It'll probably be me.* Has any anaesthetist ever had to perform open heart surgery to save a baby after both the consultant and cardiac surgery registrar dropped dead during surgery? *Can't wait to try that one!*

I am writing this on a Monday after being the consultant on call for the weekend. No, none of the above happened. In fact, nothing really happened at all. We did six operations on Saturday and eight on Sunday, all of which were minor operations on healthy children. We only anaesthetised one baby, again for relatively minor surgery. The registrars I worked with over the weekend could easily have managed all the kids by themselves. I should be thankful, but when *will* the shit hit the fan? Stay tuned …

232 – Super-Nerds

The stereotypical anaesthetist arrives in work in sweaty Lycra having steadfastly skipped the traffic on their carbon-fibre triathlon bike. They have a rudimentary shower at best before jumping into a pair of scrubs still half wet and very probably commando having forgotten to pack a clean pair of underwear. The anaesthetist, still partially out of breath, moves swiftly to the tearoom to fire up the Nespresso machine. Or for the more discerning coffee enthusiast, a dark roast from the hills near Lake Titicaca that he learned about from the local barista. This is the first of between five and seven coffees for the day. After this, a brief corridor discussion about the ridiculously long surgery from yesterday precedes the nonchalant stroll into the anaesthetic room. The laissez-faire aura of the anaesthetist is a façade and the cracks in this persona are easily spotted as he informs the registrar that they have unfortunately labelled the drug syringes horizontally and not vertically, rendering them useless. As he tosses the drugs in the bin, the looks of puzzlement on the trainee's face says it all, as they were sure the anaesthetist said the opposite last week. The anaesthetist plugs in his iPad, Bluetooth headphones, iPhone XR Plus, Apple Watch, MacBook Pro, Kindle, spare charging battery and heart-rate monitors into the sockets above the anaesthetic machine before preparing for the first case of the day. The consultant anaesthetist informs the registrar: 'You're in charge of this case. I'll do what you ask me to do.' The reluctant registrar agrees before the consultant ignores his own statement and just proceeds with his own plan anyway.

The stereotypical anaesthetist wants to appear smart in front of the nurses and surgeons, so speaks very loudly when using words such as 'compliance', 'videolayngoscope', 'target-controlled infusion' and 'ventilation strategy'. The anaesthetist always requests additional investigations when asked to anaesthetise a tricky patient, even though they'd probably be just as well simply 'cracking on'. The stereotypical anaesthetist thinks all cases are 'tricky cases', though. But the most favourite topic of conversation is the airway, their specialist subject. It is so complicated and difficult to understand that there is no point in talking to any other doctor about it, except for ENT surgeons. They get it, but everyone else just wouldn't understand.

It was during just this conversation at lunch today that I had an out-of-body experience. My mind floated up above the table and I saw myself there, with my colleagues, nattering away like excitable school children about how to manage a particular airway. It was then I realised that behind the suave air, the unflappable life-saver, lay at the core of every stereotypical anaesthetist … a super-nerd.

At the core of our specialty lies the ability to get a hollow silicone tube from the teeth of the patient, through the back of their smelly gob and down between the vocal cords. A journey of about 20 centimetres in an adult. This 20-centimetre journey (or as little as 7 cm in a teeny baby) fills us with such excitement, and occasional dread, that we can bore any other human to death in less than 60 seconds by just talking about it.

But you see, it's the fact that it's our own little journey that makes it so special, so fascinating. Every time we anaesthetise someone we use a laryngoscope, a steel device to assist us in visualising the vocal cords. No one else can see what we're doing. Sometimes we can't even see what we're doing, and this is when we dust off our toys. We have laryngoscopes of all shapes and sizes. Some have cameras attached to them. Some have cameras that can be shown on screens. Some have cameras attached to the cameras. Sometimes we use two cameras. We have straight ones. We have curved ones. We have little ones and big ones (I'm still talking about laryngoscopes, by the way).

My colleagues and I discussed a particularly difficult airway over lunch. We pretend they're all very difficult, otherwise we'd be out of a job. As we discussed the merits of using the C-MAC vs the Glidescope vs the McGrath vs the Robertshaw with BURP and a Bougie (this is all real language) a consultant surgeon sat down with us. A quick attempt to change the subject to the upcoming inclement thunderstorm was quickly shut down by us super-nerds, engrossed in our difficult airway. As I had my out-of-body experience, I saw the surgeon get up and move to the other table. None of us even noticed.

233 – Royalty

'Who is he?'

'I dunno, some lad from England, I think.'

I had spotted him in the changing room too. Sharp suit, polished shoes, nice briefcase. I presumed he was an industry rep, although they're not usually this stylish. Besides, we know the faces of most of the reps. They're usually found in the orthopaedic theatre suggesting which screw the surgeon should insert from a tray of screws the size of 20 Milk Tray boxes. *'I choose that one.' 'Very good, sir.'*

None the wiser as to who this man was, I headed off to my operating theatre for the day to get myself prepared. I overheard our two senior nurses chatting.

'He's coming today? Jesus Christ, I didn't know it was today. Look at the state of the place!'

The man downstairs, I guessed. I surveyed the room; it looked pretty much the same as always, as far as I could see. Despite this, the two nurses started frantically stuffing things in drawers and wiping down the already spotless operating table. The healthcare assistant was summoned to remove a speck of dirt found underneath the operating table.

'Who is the "he" you're all whispering about?' I asked.

'He's a surgeon from England. He's here to help Mr Foley with a case today.'

The guest surgeon – Mr Holloway. There are a couple of days like this every year. A surgeon from abroad comes for a day to either assist our consultants with a tricky, rare case or to learn a technique for themselves from our own skilled surgeons. Whether they are here to teach or be taught, the presence of Mr Holloway sparks as much panic as if the parish priest were coming over for tea in rural Ireland in the 1950s. *Jesus, Mary and Joseph – we've no fucking biscuits for the priest! He loves a Hobnob!* It's a matter of pride. Everyone is proud of the hospital they work in and no one wants visiting professionals to think our institution is in any way flawed. Time to put on the beaming smiles, laugh and shove all the shite into the cupboard for the next eight hours. It seems we're pulling out all the stops today as our guest is here to share his expertise in a particularly tricky surgical case. Obviously, no one told me he would be here, so I wasn't briefed for what I was supposed to say when asked a question by Mr Holloway. *Just stare at the ground and say thank you a lot. Do* not *make eye contact. He* hates *that.*

Mr Holloway is apparently a pretty big deal, and you'd know it judging by our surgeon's reaction when he walks into theatre to greet him. I'm starting to think it might *actually* be Elton John. Granted, there were less sequins on his suit jacket, but his glasses are cool and he's a bit of a short arse. I get cracking on the anaesthetic. I wondered if Mr Holloway witnessed me putting in the IV cannula in less than three seconds. *Can your boys do that back home?* He wasn't looking. I can overhear the small talk around me. It's making my cringe-o-meter go off the charts. I need to concentrate on what I'm doing before I spontaneously combust to remove myself from the situation. Mr Holloway seems perfectly polite, and certainly appears to enjoy the fuss. Everyone seems to be getting on just fine, provided Mr Holloway doesn't open the cupboard for all our shame to come tumbling out.

I'm provided with light entertainment throughout the case as some of the surgical equipment has chosen today to cease functioning. Our consultant surgeon sends daggers to the nurse in charge. *Please get the bloody equipment working properly.* A small bead of sweat appears on his forehead as the equipment malfunctions for the second time. Eyeball daggers to the left. Sweet and gentle chuckles to Mr Holloway on the right. 'This never happens.'

We all pat ourselves on the back as, despite the technical hiccups, the case went very smoothly. Our surgeon and Mr Holloway have completed their joint mission with the ideal outcome. Friendship, scholarship and camaraderie have all blossomed here today. Mr Holloway is invited to stay for lunch but, no, he has never been to the Guinness Storehouse so he is off on the tour before making his way back for an early evening flight. As we all wave him goodbye, like the Waltons, our belts finally loosen and we can let it all hang out again.

'I knew that camera was going to break! It's a piece of shit!' blurted out our surgical registrar.

234 – Eyes that Burn

When I was an anaesthetist in training, in every hospital I worked I always felt there was one consultant who thought I was incompetent. They would always return to theatre when the blood pressure was at its nadir, having been most fantastically perfect for the previous three hours of anaesthesia. They would watch me fail, multiple times, to place what appeared to be a straightforward IV cannula. They would witness me forget to mention an important piece of clinical information. They would sigh as I failed to successfully thread an endotracheal tube through the vocal cords. I was positive they thought I was useless. Every six months, there was one.

As least this is how I processed my shortcomings. Sometimes things are hard in medicine and I was probably missing IV cannulas or intubations no more than any other trainee. But it always felt like it was the same person I would flounder with. Did I find their presence intimidating? Was I trying too hard to make a good impression? Was I catastrophising? I still have no idea, but it was likely a combination of multiple factors. The most prominent individual factor was knowing their eyes were looking at me when I was attempting something that I knew was particularly challenging for my skill level. Sometimes you could feel the eyes warming your back as they would try, and fail, to become invisible.

I have now experienced the other side of the scenario. Being a new consultant means that I'm overbearing and interfere a lot. I'm almost certainly an unnecessary presence for the more senior trainees, thus undermining their confidence. For example, today I worked with a registrar whom I know is extremely intelligent and very capable. Today, though, it was as if it was his first day on the job. There were so many mishaps, I started to wonder if maybe I'm *that* consultant for him. I start to think that he probably gets more autonomy working with the other consultant anaesthetists, and is perfectly capable once those burning eyes are out of the room.

The poor chap had five attempts to cannulate our first child, who was ten years old, so it shouldn't really have been too taxing. The obvious veins were ripe for a needle. One miss. *No problem, there's another over there.* A second miss. *It can be tricky in this age group.* A third. *Ok, really make sure you pick a decent one this time.* A fourth. *Silence.* A fifth miss. *Ok let's swap places, I'll put one in.* As I managed to place the cannula with ease, I felt bad. In those situations, as a trainee, you hope, with all your heart, that the consultant also makes a balls of it. Praying for the consultant to fail was a regular feature of my training.

After more missed cannulas and a missed endotracheal tube, I began to realise that I should probably just leave him be. So, I removed myself from the theatre as the next child arrived. I did a few laps of the theatre department before returning. I half expected him to still be looking for a vein but no, the cannula was in, endotracheal tube was in, the surgeons were scrubbed. Surgery had begun. Wow, he did that fast. No pressure from the lurking consultant.

240 – Dad Jokes

Everyone has gone through the change. It's a fact of life. There comes a point when kids switch from thinking their parents are rib-ticklingly funny to being painfully embarrassing dimwits. I can't pinpoint the exact moment that it happened to me, but it was certainly somewhere in the early teenage years, probably coinciding with that troubling part of childhood where you start to care how you are perceived by your peers. Parents just aren't cool at that stage. I see it when the teenagers arrive in theatre accompanied by a parent who is stiff with fear of the operation their precious not-so-small-any-more baby is about to have. The teenager, on the other hand, is more uncomfortable with the presence of their mother so close to them when they have no underpants on under their hospital gown. The quicker I can knock them out, the better – for them.[50]

I have discovered an anomaly to this parent–child comedy relationship, though. In this strange arrangement, the parent (99 per cent of the time it's the dad) woefully misjudges their young child's anxiety levels relating to their impending operation. Rather than trying to make them feel better, Dad repeatedly cracks glaringly inappropriate jokes about the operation, expecting their usually receptive child to find it hilarious. They do not. As the child gets more terrified by the subject matter of Dad's insensitive jokes, Dad repeats the jokes and stares at me, the anaesthetist, in the hope that I take his side and give him a hearty chuckle. Unbeknownst to Dad, his jokes are actually making my job infinitely more difficult and the poor kid now has no trust for anyone in authority and certainly not the man who is about to launch at them with a gas mask.

---

50 I can assure any parents reading, whose teenagers are currently less talkative than a cinder block, that this phase passes and parents become hilarious and good company again once the twenties hit.

Example one occurred a number of years ago in Australia, during an orthopaedic list. Many fractured bones do not need surgery, they simply require the offending body part to be placed in a rigid cast. The rigid casts, though rarely 'plaster of Paris' these days, still have to be removed with special equipment. Ok, it's not that special. I'll be blunt – it's a fucking gigantic saw. Now the saw (it actually vibrates) has a safety mechanism whereby it only saws through the cast and no further, but obviously, for the uninformed child, this is possibly the most terrifying thing they have ever experienced in their life. It takes less than 20 seconds to remove a cast with the saw and it is in no way painful. Therefore, casts are removed wherever the patient happens to be, anywhere from the A&E to the outpatients to the day unit.

A young kid was added onto our operating list that day for a 'cast removal under general anaesthesia'. I had never seen this before – there had to be a story. The orthopaedic nurse did not disappoint when she informed me that the child had gone 'absolutely fucking ballistic' when attempts were made to saw off the cast on the day unit. Unfortunately, it seems the father thought he would announce that the doctors couldn't fix the broken arm, so they were going to have to saw it clean off. Most adults would be somewhat apprehensive at the prospect of a stranger taking a saw anywhere near their arm, let alone a small child. No amount of talking, bribery or coercion could get this kid to play ball after this idiotic joke. A large dose of sedation didn't do the trick either. The way the kid saw it, the drugs were the prelude to the upcoming amputation. Next stop, general anaesthesia. A second sedative allowed us to sneak an intravenous cannula into the child's hand. In case of any further slips of the tongue, Dad was substituted with Mum, who joined us in theatre, where we gave our patient the briefest of general anaesthetics to get that pesky cast off, limb still intact.

Example two occurred today. What is it with dads and chopping things off? Are they all from the Freddy Krueger generation? Is this what terrified them as kids, and they want their little snowflakes to suffer too? I can't understand it. You won't need to be a Mensa member to guess what young Jamie thought would be cut off when I tell you he was in theatre for a circumcision. Jamie walked into the anaesthetic room like a lost lamb, if lost lambs walked upright cupping their genitals in two hands while gingerly entering an operating theatre. Dad followed behind, beaming from ear to ear, whispering, 'They're going to cut it off!' Dad looked at me expecting a high five, a wink or a dig in the ribs or a whatever else he wanted after telling his son he was going to have his fucking dick cut off. I did not join in, turned my back on Dad and went about correcting Jamie's expectations of this minor surgical procedure. He finally took his hands away from his crotch as I explained that, no, his penis would not be all gone and that I would ensure he had no pain when he woke up. Dad, looking deflated that I was such a party-pooper, slumped into a chair and said no more.

247 – The Key to Anaesthesia

We get a lot of children with autism through the theatre department. Some of these kids have a formal diagnosis, while others have been 'diagnosed' by their parents, who inform us that their child is 'on the spectrum'. Autism, or 'autistic spectrum disorder', is very much a spectrum.[51] Some children will have fairly mild foibles and idiosyncrasies in their behaviour while others can be really quite disabled and have severe difficulty in communicating. It is, in essence, a developmental disorder characterised by difficulties in communicating (both verbal and non-verbal), socialising and often with repetitive and restrictive behaviour. The phrase autism is derived from 'auto-ism', or being within oneself. On the more severe end of the spectrum, children with autism may have aggressive tendencies,

---

51 It's not caused by vaccinations either – don't be ridiculous.

self-injurious behaviour or hyperactive behaviour. Repetitive patterns of behaviour can provide comfort to the children and thus breaking their routines can result in distress and significant anxiety.

The diagnosis of autism comes from very specific diagnostic criteria. While some children certainly fall within the diagnostic criteria, others do not, but still somehow end up with a label of 'autism' and the unfortunate stigma that still goes with it. This can be the case when a child has a multitude of other medical problems that contribute to learning or behavioural problems. It is easy to label all behavioural problems as being 'autistic'. This is not something we, or child psychiatrists, do, but can happen in the community. It is a very important distinction to make, as early intervention strategies for truly autistic children are very important for their development and can be considerably different for children who have behavioural problems that are not due to autism. Not all behavioural problems are due to autism and not all children with autism have severe behavioural problems.

Children with autism frequently appear on the same operating lists: dental surgery, ENT surgery and for MRI scans. When you meet a severely autistic child, you can see why this makes complete sense. It can be difficult for parents to maintain good oral hygiene in their autistic child as getting access to brush their teeth or encourage them to do so is troublesome. Similarly, a severely autistic child will not let you examine their ears in any great detail and if an MRI is required for any indication, you can think again if you expect someone with anxiety or behavioural problems to lie still for 30 minutes in a cold and claustrophobic MRI machine. When considering all this, anaesthetists have a lot of interactions with children who have autism. The process of anaesthetising some of this group is very challenging. Often, they will require heavy premedication to the point where they are in a deep sleep even before coming to the operating theatre. Breaking their cycle of behaviour and their expectations of the day does not come easily.

It helps (me, anyway) to ask the parents what comforting behaviours their child likes to use when in a stressful situation and to do our best to allow this to continue to happen. On occasion, incorporating this comforting act into our anaesthetic plan can eliminate the need for premedication and it can be very surprising, as it was today. An older boy with autism, Craig, was listed for an MRI. On reading his clinical notes, it was clear he had severe autism. He was non-verbal and was not independent in any way, meaning that his parents would dress him and carry out simple tasks for him. As I read more, I thought this would be a challenging anaesthetic. I made my way over to the bedside to introduce myself to Craig and his parents. He was lying in the bed gazing at a set of keys. Not one, not two, but three different sets of keys were all collected in a little pile. One set was being scrupulously investigated, the other two merely waiting their turn. He glanced up at me standing at the end of the bed and immediately got out and onto his feet. He hurried over to me and plunged his hands into my scrub pockets. Within seconds, he had retrieved my keys and triumphantly annexed them to his growing mound of keys. Counting all his keys, he probably had access to property worth over €1,000,000 at this stage. His mother didn't need to explain that collecting keys was Craig's comforting, repetitive behaviour.[52] His mother told me that if we just permitted him to collect some keys and keep them nearby, he would easily let us place a mask over his nose and mouth to be anaesthetised. I had my doubts, but I took her word for it.

As I waited for the MRI staff to do their safety checks, I explained to the nurses what would probably happen and to just, well, let it happen. We gathered in the anaesthetic room and waited. A couple of minutes later, Craig walked in clutching three sets of keys – his father's, his mother's and our porter's. Before he would climb onto the bed, he again whipped mine clean out of my pocket before

---

52 Or a precursor to a life of kleptomania.

inspecting the pockets of all three nurses present. He found one more set and then stole the anaesthetic registrar's keys right out of his hands. Six sets of keys should do the trick. His mother gave me the nod to start. Still apprehensive of what might happen, I gently placed the mask onto his nose first, then down over his mouth. He didn't even flinch. Twenty seconds later, Craig was asleep.[53]

248 – The Theatre of Theatre

When a patient is on cardiopulmonary bypass (CPB) to facilitate open heart surgery, the heart and lungs are redundant. The CPB machine takes over the work that these critical organs usually perform. The heart is stopped with a 'cardioplegia' solution and we turn off the ventilator. It allows the surgeons to open the heart and operate on a still, blood-free heart. On CPB, we hand control of the patient over to the perfusionist, who runs the CPB machine, keeps the patient asleep and manages their physiology. All of this makes us anaesthetists also fairly redundant when we are on CPB, aside from adjusting the height of the table for the surgeon. *Ten years of training to be a bed technician.* The process of separating the patient from CPB back to their own heart and lungs at the end of the surgery can be a very turbulent phase of surgery, so often we spend the time the patient is on CPB preparing for the transition.

The time spent on CPB during an operation varies depending on the complexity of surgery. Needless to say, we have to entertain ourselves somehow during long runs on CPB. On bypass today, I took the opportunity to do some paperwork and sat in the corner of the theatre with my laptop. Despite our super-slick operating theatre, we still have little to no Wi-Fi in the hospital. To counter this, being a slick older millennial myself, I turned on the personal

---

53 The keys did not come into the scanning room with him – the radiology staff made me write that in case they got in trouble.

hotspot on my phone to tether some internet to my laptop. I click on the little Wi-Fi tab on the laptop to find 'Colin Black's iPhone'. Being in an operating theatre, I expected my phone to be the only Wi-Fi signal available, but not so.

There were a couple of generic, indecipherable names:

VM U87368
Printer_4533

But below, to my delight:

Pretty-wi-for-a-fi-guy[54]

I sat up in my chair, intrigued. *Who is this person?* A game of real-life 'Guess Who?' was on the cards here – what a way to spend a few hours on bypass! Due to the implicit gender profiling of the Wi-Fi name, I ruled out the women. I scanned the room. There were three surgeons: the professor of cardiac surgery, his male senior registrar and female junior registrar – I flip down her 'Guess Who' avatar. There were two perfusionists, both male. There was an anaesthetic nurse, female – flip, gone. There was a scrub nurse – female, gone – and three circulating nurses, one male and two female – rapid-fire flip-flip. Having watched too much *Mindhunter* on Netflix, I decided I was going to have to profile my Offspring fan to further investigate:

Aged 32–45
Once dyed hair peroxide blond
Still thinks The Offspring is good

_____

54 For the connoisseur of late nineties pop-punk music, I don't need to tell you this is a clever play on The Offspring song 'Pretty Fly (for a White Guy)'.

Tried to skateboard as a teenager
Still wears Vans and is delighted by their recent resurgence
Had at least one piercing
Considered becoming a full-blown Emo
Is computer savvy, as they would have had to change their
    Wi-Fi network name manually

I studied the profile and realised that I fit at least four of the criteria (not telling you which) but I rule myself out because, well, it's my game. So, I'm left with five other men. I rule out the circulating nurse as he's no older than 25. Sadly, I also rule out the professor of cardiac surgery, as I think he may not fit the age criteria either (treading carefully). This leaves me with three distinct possibilities: the cardiac surgery registrar and the two perfusionists. I try to picture them all as younger men with peroxide blond hair and lip piercings. Not helpful. I try to recall if I have seen any of them wearing a pair of Vans in the changing rooms. Not to the best of my recollection. I scan their faces and ears for evidence of old piercings. Can't spot anything from where I'm sitting and to go in for a closer look might be weird. I don't know anyone's age but at a guess only one of the perfusionists really fits the bill. *Is it you? Will I ever know?* I click on the Wi-Fi network and am asked to enter a password: 'perfusion'. No luck, I'm out of ideas.

Let me just re-think this. The professor did work in America, probably when The Offspring was gaining popularity in the late 90s. Is that an old piercing I see in his ear? *Is it?*

253 – Assume the Position

Patients are placed in various positions to facilitate surgery. It's a good thing they're under anaesthesia when this happens as some positions are not so flattering. Some positions are more natural than others. The 'supine' position is most common – lying on your back with arms by your side. You can perform most surgeries in the supine position. The 'lateral' position is on the side, much like how you would position yourself if sleeping on your side. This is the position required for some operations on the chest or back. It gets a bit odd after that. The 'prone' position is lying face down and, as you can imagine, is necessary for operations on the back, neck or bum. Next is the 'lithotomy' position, a variation of supine, except that your knees may be drawn towards your chest with the legs hoisted up into stirrups, like the position commonly used in labour. Lithotomy is needed for urological, gynaecological or some rectal operations. Maybe the strangest position is the sitting position, used rarely in neurosurgery only. It is natural, I guess, except for the fact that you're unconscious in the sitting position, making it a bit disconcerting for the staff. Once you are in whatever position you need to be in, the operating table itself can be manoeuvred. Head down is called 'Trendelenberg', after a West German surgeon. Head up is 'reverse Trendelenberg', after an East German surgeon. These are not sex positions, or at least not that I am aware of. The bed can also be tilted side to side. All these variations give any number of combinations.

Exposure of one's rear-end is almost a given. Patients are often concerned by this as they clutch the back of their hospital gown on the way to surgery to avoid their bare arse flapping in the breeze. Some insist on keeping underwear on (as they are entitled to do if they so wish) when having anaesthesia induced, despite the full knowledge that they are coming off almost as soon as we move into theatre for most (not all) operations. It wouldn't make any sense to have no pants on for ear surgery. Having an exposed bum was the primary concern of a friend of mine who had to go for emergency back surgery. She called me with grave concerns. Her attention was not on the fact that she was in severe pain with a surgical ailment, it was the fact that the operating theatre staff would all see her bum. 'Oh. My. God. Colin, will they all see my ass?' Needless to say, everyone in theatre has seen everything so many times that we really don't flinch at the sight of any naked body.

Positioning adults can be hard and great care must be taken. If you think a 120 kg man is heavy when awake, try moving one when they are fully anaesthetised. It can feel like shifting a baby elephant and takes up to eight people to do so correctly without the patient, or the lifters, getting injured. Positioning kids is obviously a lot easier; where it takes eight people to move a large man, it takes one hand to move a baby. I have observed, though, that there is one position that seems to cause frequent frustration and cursing in the operating theatre – lithotomy. Where in adult hospitals all over the country legs are flung in the air for hundreds of urological and gynaecological operations every day, this is a lot less frequent in kids. In fact, gynaecological operations are almost non-existent in kids and urological operations requiring lithotomy are also relatively rare.

Every time lithotomy is required, it looks to me like the surgeons are positioning a patient for the first time. Watching them piece together the equipment needed for the stirrups to sit correctly is like watching a four-year-old build a scale model of Notre Dame out of Lego. Our surgeons today finally made inroads after ten minutes. Ready! Not so: the senior nurse pointed out that they put the pieces together backwards. Further fiddling ensued and, finally, all the pieces appeared to be pointing in the right direction, ready for our toddler's legs to be lifted into them.

Lithotomy position takes a bit of care to ensure the patient doesn't injure themselves while asleep. Poor positioning can put pressure on muscles, nerves or joints, and obviously you yourself can't shift position when you are anaesthetised. Trying to make the unnatural natural is challenging. In adults, the equipment fits most people nicely, and thanks to the stiffer hips of those over 30 the legs usually come to a fairly comfortable-looking position. Kids, though, are super-mobile. I watch our surgeons place the two legs gently into the stirrups and let go. Both legs flop and fall wildly out to either side to assume a frog-like position. They make adjustments and try again. This time, one leg goes out and the other flops inwards, with both knees now leaning in the same direction. I hear audible sighs. More adjustments to the height of the stirrups and the position of the feet. Now both knees turn inwards, almost knocking into each other. After 15 minutes I hear the surgeon curse.

After two more failed attempts, the stirrups are promptly removed from the operating table. The consultant surgeon instructs his registrar and SHO to grab a leg each and just hold them in position for him. The operation takes three minutes.

254 – White Lies

Here are some white lies that I encounter as an anaesthetist.

'We're just leaving the ward' – all staff nurses

When we are ready in theatre, someone will 'send' for the next patient. This is usually a phone call to the ward. We sent for a baby today at 2.15 p.m. (having given the ward warning 20 minutes prior). The baby was situated, to be fair, in the furthest ward from the operating theatre, hence the advance warning. It can take about three minutes to walk there, or five if you're really just out for a stroll. 2.30 p.m., we call again.

'Has baby O'Brien left the ward?'

'Sorry, we're just leaving the ward now.'

We get the theatre prepared for the imminent arrival. We turn up the temperature for a small baby, we prepare tiny little syringes of cute little baby drugs. We chat and have a bit of banter to pass the time. The laughing stops at 2.40 p.m. when there is no baby. At 2.45 p.m., we call again.

'Sorry, we've been waiting for 30 minutes now. Where is baby O'Brien?'

'We got delayed. We're just leaving the ward now.'

A little steam puffs out of everyone's ears. This is annoying. Baby O'Brien is not the last case on the list, so we need to get moving. We sit in silence this time. Ten minutes pass, no baby. I start to wonder if I was mistaken. Maybe that ward is much further away than I thought? I expect to see a dishevelled nurse crawling up the corridor, baby O'Brien cradled in her arms. She is cut and scratched. Blood oozes from her ears. Her clothes are torn. Her lips are cracked. She wipes the snow out of her hair to whisper, 'We lost the mother.' She uses her last ounce of strength to present us with an unharmed baby O'Brien, before dying in front of us.

3 p.m., we call again – this time I call, with my (pathetic) authoritative voice.

'Hi, excuse me, this is Dr Black, the consultant anaesthetist. We have a full theatre team here waiting for baby O'Brien for the last 45 minutes. This is a ridiculous waste of everyone's time. Where is the baby?'

'Baby O'Brien has left the ward.'

LIFT-OFF: ELVIS HAS LEFT THE BUILDING. Disappointingly, there is no snow, no bites from a sabre-toothed tiger or no tale of interest to account for the mysterious 45 minutes of lost time. I do my best to give a 'filthy' to the nurse. She smiles. God, I'm pathetic.

'This is a quick, five-minute job' – all surgeons

This is the same cognitive bias that goes with driving tests. Apparently, most people think they are above-average drivers, despite the fact that this defies the law of averages – half of you must be below average at driving. Surgery must be a super-duper enjoyable pastime if you are the one performing it, but it is pretty tedious for us to be watching most of the time. I've only met a handful of surgeons who are entirely realistic about how fast or slow they operate. Fast isn't always better, by the way (although it does get us home quicker).

This white lie usually appears in the late afternoon (or occasionally approaching midnight). It's 4.05 p.m.; theatres are supposed to be finished at 5 p.m. The surgeon was a bit slower than usual for one or two of the other cases (although they'll blame slow anaesthesia) and now we're under pressure to get the last case done. Is there time? It doesn't look like a quick one. The surgeon looks at me. I look at the nurse in charge. The surgeon looks at the nurse in charge. Really, the nurse in charge is the boss. 'This is a quick, five-minute job,' vomits the consultant surgeon, almost reflexively.

We take the plunge, the patient arrives. We minimise our anaesthetic faff time to get the patient anaesthetised and ready, and off we go. The surgeon begins. It's 4.20 p.m. I glance over the drapes at 4.40 p.m.; things seem to be going steady. 4.50 p.m. arrives; I should really hear them asking for sutures to close the skin now. The surgeon appears concerned, but says nothing. 5 p.m. – it's happened again. We all fell for it. Such fools we are! Duped, yet again!

'Colin, this is a little trickier than I thought it would be.'

'Mmmmm-hhhhmmmm.'

I send the registrar home and settle in for the unknown. How long will we be here for? The nurse in charge gives me one of those looks, like it was my fault. *Dammit, we all agreed to this!*

'Oh yeah, everything's fine up here' – all anaesthetists

I can't really reveal the little white lies from other groups without admitting that, yes, even the anaesthetists can't be trusted. We sit at the head of the operating table, near the patient's head and close to our ventilator and monitors. We have an abundance of information at our fingertips that we interpret, in real time, to give us an idea of 'how well' the patient is doing.

It is true that if the anaesthetist panics, then everyone else panics too. We are supposed to be the calming influence. From the surgeon's perspective, from where they operate, the less they can see the anaesthetist in their peripheral vision, behind the drapes, the better. If they can't see us, then they reason that the anaesthetist must be calmly sitting in their chair playing *Candy Crush*.

The anaesthetist's annoying cranium only appears over the top of the drapes for two reasons: to see why the fucking fuck the fucking operation is taking so fucking long, or because they are somewhat concerned for the patient's status. We stand up to get drugs, to adjust the ventilator, to give more fluid, to ask the nurse to bring blood. The surgeon can sense which of the two scenarios it is; they usually know if the operation is going on longer than planned. If they sense the second, more worrying scenario then it is followed by an, 'Is everything ok up there?' To which we reply with our stock answer, 'Oh yeah, everything's fine up here.' At which point we slowly turn the monitor away from the surgeon's gaze as we quietly sort out the problem.

I was once in theatre with a consultant anaesthetist, as a trainee. As we were preparing to commence surgery, I witnessed the blood pressure of the patient plummet, while their heart rate started to rocket. The consultant had just injected a dose of antibiotics. He peered under the drapes to inspect the patient's skin and noticed a widespread rash. This was a barn-door anaphylactic reaction to the antibiotic, a genuine and life-threatening emergency. If it happened outside the hospital, a patient's airway could rapidly close over and they could die. But, under anaesthesia, although the airway is already protected with an ETT, it is still a genuine emergency. The consultant gently turned the monitor away from the rest of the theatre before turning to me. He whispered, 'The patient is having an anaphylactic reaction. We don't want to cause any panic.' He casually treated the patient with some adrenalin and steroids and the reaction settled before the surgeon had even made an incision. No one was any the wiser.[55]

255 – A Bolt from the Blue (Light)

Since becoming a consultant, I've become even more acutely aware of just how unhealthy and stressful shift work can be for healthcare professionals. The vast majority of this sort of work for a doctor occurs during your training, from intern to SHO to registrar. The reason I am more acutely aware of it is because I don't have to do it any more, and I can literally feel the difference in my health. It's blatantly obvious to me now. It makes me appreciate the work our registrars do and simultaneously curse the rota system we have, especially as doctors.

When I began as an intern, 36-hour shifts were the norm. We would arrive for work on a Monday morning, do a 'normal day' of work (nothing 'normal' about a 7 a.m. to 7 p.m. working day) before picking up the on-call pager and spending the next 12 hours on call in the hospital and managing any issues arising. We might possibly crash for a mere two hours of broken sleep throughout the night, and before we knew it, it was Tuesday morning, and we would begin another 'normal' zombified day of work.

During my senior house officer years, shifts were limited to 'only' 24 hours, allowing us at least to collapse into bed the following morning at home. We would do this up to three times per week. This working pattern was manageable when young and full of beans. Personally, it only started to take its toll on me as a registrar. On-call life as a registrar is very much dependent on the specialty you choose. For example, some registrars do no on-call at all (e.g. dermatology), some can do their on-call from home, only coming

---

55 Of course, he did disclose this information to both surgeon and patient afterwards and the appropriate referrals were made to an allergy expert.

to hospital for emergencies (e.g. ENT surgery, plastic surgery), some are permitted to be at home but often don't bother as they're too busy (e.g. general surgery) and others are obliged to be in-house at all times (e.g. anaesthesia, intensive care, general medicine).

In anaesthesia training, we spend a lot of time working in intensive care. At night, you tend to the sickest patients in the hospital, usually alone, as well as being the go-to person for the wards and ED, if anyone else decides they want to try to die during the night. The night consists of constant alarms piercing your skull. It's unrelenting telephone calls from wards or other doctors. It's making urgent life-and-death clinical decisions repeatedly, all night long. When you do get a chance to put your head down and rest, the phone rings again, or the cardiac arrest pager goes off. You constantly have surges of adrenalin in response to the next clinical emergency. You wake bolt upright every time the pager goes off, even if it is for something trivial, as you expect to have to run to the ward to start CPR on someone. Try going back to sleep with that adrenalin in your veins causing your heart to vibrate in your chest and pupils to dilate. Some anaesthesia doctors unfortunately drop the training programme after working in the ICU.

I didn't think it affected my health until my last long rotation in intensive care. I began getting thundering headaches during each shift on call, the kind where you can feel your brain pulsating. At one point I got a migraine aura for the first time, and I couldn't see during a night shift. I checked my blood pressure – 160/90. This is high enough to begin anti-hypertensive medication. I would check it when not in work. 120/80. Then in the middle of the night, sleep-deprived having been woken bolt upright, I would check again. 160/90. As soon as I graduated to senior registrar and no longer had to work ICU shifts, my blood pressure normalised. The rise in blood pressure is natural and necessary in a critical scenario. Your adrenalin prepares you for fight-or-flight. It focuses the mind. What is unhealthy is a surge in adrenalin in response to something innocuous such as a phone call or a bleeping pager. Pavlov's dogs again.

I was reminded of the feeling last night as I was on call. As a consultant I am now on call in my own bed. We don't have much activity overnight in the operating theatre in a children's hospital. This has afforded me a full night's sleep on every single one of my on-calls since I began eight months ago. Last night, however, the phone rang deep into the night at 2.30 a.m. The familiar feeling. I sat bolt upright, with my heart pounding, even before I answered the phone.

It's the unknown that's frightening. What is the request on the other end of the line? Is there a child dying when I am 20 minutes from the hospital? Is there a baby bleeding terribly after heart surgery? Is there a huge road accident and we must rush to theatre to save a child's life? On this occasion, I did have to go back to the hospital in the cold, dark of night. The operation was not as acute as I feared, but acute enough to be happy that the burst of adrenalin had zipped my senses back into focus. I returned to my own bed at 4.30 a.m. and didn't sleep a wink for the rest of the night.

268 – The Elusive Vein

I won't lie, it's nice to be considered an 'expert' at something. Most of the time. We are the 'experts' at IV cannulation which is only, I confess, partially true. Yes, we can put tiny cannulas into tiny babies, but let's not forget that, for the most part, they are lying perfectly still under anaesthesia when we do so. Being successful at the same task with an awake, wriggling, screaming baby and terrified parents is where the true skill lies.

Cannulating awake adults is easy, and awake children, if they are compliant, is also relatively easy. Cannulating anyone who is both awake and utterly terrified is most certainly not. The anxiety in the eyes of some kids coming to theatre is obvious. I start to feel the pressure when a parent begins with, 'There's no need to be scared. This man is the expert. He can do it so quickly.' *Hold on a second there.* There are a few parts to a successful cannulation – poke the needle through the skin (this is the most painful part), hitting a vein and then sliding the plastic cannula off the needle into the vein itself. This is all before securing the bloody thing (no pun intended) before the child pulls it out. I feel the pressure for the second time when, after the needle pokes through the skin, the parent (or sometimes my very own anaesthetic nurse – they should know better!) declares to the child that it's all over. I have to remind them that it is most certainly not over until I can see that little flash of scarlet blood in the chamber indicating that I've hit a vein.

Teenagers coming for scoliosis correction are almost universally anxious. They are gaining independence, very self-aware and not always pleased to be coming to have major surgery on their spine when, in reality, their curvy spine may not even bother them all that much at the present time. Put all those things together and you get a group of frightened and coy adolescents, like our patient today. As I introduced myself to him, the first thing he declared was that under no circumstances was he having a mask induction, after his previous traumatic experience as a small child.

'That's not a problem,' I said. 'I prefer to put a needle in the hand when people are your age.'

'I'm really scared of needles.'

This is a pretty typical reply, but I got the sense that he really meant it. To counter this, I prescribed him a premedication and applied some gel that numbs the skin to minimise the pain of the cannula. I knew he had arrived in theatre when I heard audible sobs travelling along the corridor. With tears streaming down his face, he was trembling like a leaf. Our premedication appeared not to have been too successful today. To distract him as the nurses placed some monitoring on, I asked him what he was scared about. The needle. Always the needle. Then came the dreaded words out of his mother's mouth: 'This man is the expert, he won't have any problems and it will be over so fast.' Three blatant lies but what can I do but agree and nod my head.

Veins go into hiding in the nervous hand. As I gently took both his hands to have a look at the situation, they were clammy, cold and mottled. Not a vein in sight. All sure-fire signs that his 'fight-or-flight' response had taken hold and now he had adrenalin coursing through his veins. This was confirmed as I heard the beep of the monitoring. I didn't need to look to know his heart rate was well over 100 beats per minute. He hyperventilated and puffed and panted, sobbing intermittently. I applied the tourniquet in the desperate hope a blue vein would suddenly appear. Nothing. We distracted him some more, asking about school. His heart rate slowed briefly but would pick up almost instantly if I even glanced at his hand. At last, a sliver of a skinny vein appeared. There would be one attempt at this before a complete meltdown, of this I was sure.

I rolled his hand into a fist and told him to look at his mum. I gently disinfected the skin and reached for the needle. A deep breath for all involved and … plunge. A shriek and a cry shook the room despite our numbing gel. No blood in the chamber. I begin to sweat. Mum glances over and chimes in with the second worst thing to say – 'It's all over, it's in!' *Ugh, please be quiet, you're not helping.* I readjust the needle under the skin and redirect it once more before another advance towards the elusive vein. A flash of scarlet in the chamber. *Thank fuck for that.* I give myself a second to be sure before I slide the plastic tube into the vein and withdraw the needle. It looks good. He looks over as I finally declare that the worst is over, and he is palpably relieved. I can sense the pounding in his chest started to abate. His breathing slows down. I immediately give him some intravenous sedation which takes effect almost instantly. He is finally ready to be anaesthetised. I feel like I've done a day's worth of work even with this elementary task, but we are just getting started on an eight-hour operation.

269 – A Healthy Baby?

My wife is pregnant with our first baby. I didn't see how it was relevant to mention up until this point but today we went for our anatomical scan. This is the antenatal scan at around 20 weeks' gestation that looks, in depth, at the anatomy of the foetus with a view to diagnosing any major problems that can be picked up at this stage. It doesn't rule out everything but can certainly be very reassuring if it all looks normal. The rate of congenital anomaly is somewhere around 2 per cent overall, but less in a low-risk pregnancy (<1 per cent). The degree of severity of a congenital anomaly is spread across a very broad range, from something causing little or no disability to other anomalies that are fatal.

I never really thought about this much until my wife fell pregnant. I now realise that I suffer from a serious cognitive bias due to the fact that I work in a children's hospital. I had resigned myself to the fact that our unborn child will most certainly have a major congenital abnormality. In the last few weeks I have been ruminating about which organ will be affected. Will it have a serious cardiac condition? Will it have an abnormal brain? Will the abdominal contents be lying outside its little body? I had a sort of league table in my head of which would be most preferable and which I would be wishing against. The source of my bias lies in the fact that the chances of a child with a major congenital anomaly requiring surgery are infinitely higher than a healthy child requiring surgery. This is evident every single day in our operating theatre as we anaesthetise children frequently for surgery to correct, cure or palliate these major problems. Therefore, the majority of the children I meet in work have some congenital anomaly.

I won't lie, I was shitting myself as we sat in the waiting room. Although our record would clearly state both my wife and I are doctors, the sonographer didn't appear to notice. Probably for the best. As I sat there quivering, the scan began at the head. *There is a head and a brain, excellent.* Onto the face where she would look for a cleft lip or palate. No evidence of such but the anaesthetist in me was looking at the lower jaw, the mandible. *Is that a bit small?* A small mandible suggests a difficult intubation and can be associated with syndromes like Treacher–Collins or Pierre–Robin. No time to think; we were onto the limbs. There were four of them and the measurements seemed in keeping with the estimated dates. Some major orthopaedic anomalies can be diagnosed at this point. Next to the abdomen. *Bowels are in the belly, not outside.* Major abnormalities of the abdominal wall include diagnoses such as omphalocele or gastroschisis where all or some of the abdominal contents lie outside of the body. She showed us the diaphragm, beautifully intact. The diaphragm separates the thorax from the abdomen. A defect here can cause a major anomaly called a diaphragmatic hernia where the abdominal contents move into the thorax and impede growth of a lung. She measured the amount of amniotic fluid, which was in the normal range. This indicates that the foetus is able to swallow fluid and also pee it out, reducing the chances of oesophageal or urinary problems.

Now onto the heart. I sat up in anticipation. With so much of my training geared at congenital heart disease, I most certainly had a league table of which anomaly would be easily repaired and which could be fatal. My eyes focused. 'Show me the four chambers of the heart!', I screamed in my head. There appeared to be four, some relief. She labelled the two atria and two ventricles. *Well, there must be transposition of the great arteries.* Transposition of the great arteries (TGA) is where the two major arteries from the heart are attached to the wrong ventricle, meaning the blood is not going where it is supposed to. She scanned and labelled the structures – LVOT and Ao (left ventricular outflow tract and aorta respectively). This is normal. Then RVOT and PA (right ventricular outflow tract and pulmonary artery respectively). This is also normal. *OK, well there must be a large VSD, so.* A ventricular septal defect (VSD) is an abnormal connection between the two ventricles. She turned on the Doppler signal which indicates which way the blood was moving. All in the right direction. All of a sudden the ultrasound probe was down on the abdomen again. *Was that it? It was all normal?!*

Next, we examined the urological system. My wife perked up. There were two kidneys of normal size and below them sat the distinct lovely trigone of a bladder, like a black triangle floating in the middle of the screen. We looked away as the sonographer determined the sex of the foetus, although I know we both tried to have a sneaky look earlier in the scan. A normal urological system was followed by a normal spine. It was all normal. I had not really prepared for this unexpected diagnosis of a normal, healthy foetus. What is the strange diagnosis? It was rare in my books. I was at a bit of a loss. All that emotional preparation was directed towards receiving a devastating diagnosis and how we would cope with such news.

As I read the ultrasound report that essentially said 'normal' in every box, I spotted the disclaimer. In bold, at the bottom of the page, 'A normal ultrasound cannot rule out a congenital anomaly.' Having partially adapted to the crazy idea of having a healthy baby, this was shunting me back towards my cognitive bias. *Don't get too excited by this 'normal' scan.*

We sat down with the consultant obstetrician, who took one brief glance at the report and announced that it all looked grand, like he does many times a day. Despite this, I still held on to the possibility that things could change and did not get excited. It was only until he said in passing 'the anatomy doesn't change' that this became real to me. Why am I being so unsure? *Of course the fucking anatomy doesn't change, Colin!* Of course the brain won't just disappear. Of course the great arteries can't just switch over to the wrong position at the last minute. Of course kidneys stay attached to the bladder. Why, for someone generally so rational, was I being so irrational?

A career in paediatric practice has me primed for the worst. I was only now, in that room, coming to terms with the very high probability that our baby will be healthy. Of course, the ultrasound can't determine any genetic abnormality, but it certainly appears that our potato-sized human looks healthy. But there will always be that sliver of doubt in my head until delivery day.

274 – Performance Anxiety

I have been called back to the hospital at 10 p.m. to anaesthetise a five-year-old girl with a bad supracondylar fracture. This is a fairly common fracture just above the elbow in kids. These fractures can disrupt the nerves and blood supply to the arm, therefore they often need urgent repair. The surgeon uttered the golden words, 'neuro-vascular compromise', and I was on the way in.

Knowing how long it takes for a child to arrive in theatre directly from the ED (about as long as it took J. R. R. Tolkien to write *The Lord of the Rings*, the time it took to build the Great Wall of China or about twice as long as it would take to count all the grains of sand in the Sahara Desert), I tell the registrar to send for the child when I'm still at home. I'm about a 20-minute drive from the hospital, and it would be a miracle if the child were there, in theatre, on my arrival. My suspicions are correct as I land in theatre and there is no sign of anything happening. There are also three nurses who have come in from home. The orthopaedic registrar has also called in the orthopaedic consultant, so by 10.30 p.m. there are seven of us all twiddling our thumbs for the grand arrival. *Maybe they are actually writing a sequel to* The Lord of the Rings. We all look at each other, becoming blearier-eyed and impatient.

Eventually, at 10.45 p.m., a tired-looking little Russian girl, Katrin, arrives with her equally tired-looking mother. We quickly ascertain that, although her mother speaks good English, Katrin doesn't speak any at all. As we describe the plan, Mum nods but

Katrin begins to look intently at her. After attaching all our monitoring and completing our final checks, I reach for our tray of drugs and approach the cannula in Katrin's hand. She quickly turns to Mum, whimpering, and whispers in her ear. There is some mumbling in Russian. I put the tray down. Mum announces that Katrin needs to go to the toilet. 10.55 p.m. Our Polish nurse quickly replies, 'No, she can wait, it's no problem.' I admire her desire to press on and get us all back to our beds. No messing. But Katrin looks upset and insists. The toilets are back up the corridor and it would be a tricky manoeuvre for Mum to get her off the bed and into the toilet considering she won't let anyone move her arm for the pain. A basin is produced and promptly thrust under the blanket. Mum gently lifts up Katrin's backside and dumps her in the basin, under the sheets. We wait.

10.57 p.m. – Katrin gazes dead ahead at the wall, supported on the left by her mum and the right by a nurse. The anaesthetic team lean against the window behind. The orthopaedic team to the far left flick through the x-rays of her fracture and discuss their surgical plan. No pee-pee.

10.58 p.m. – Katrin fixes her gaze on the clock on the wall and appears to be squinting slightly in an attempt to urinate. No pee-pee.

11.00 p.m. – Katrin's bum is still in the basin. There appears to be no end to this pee. We must be ready for a basin change at this point.

11.01 p.m. – The anaesthetic team get shifty and make eye contact with the nurse. She shakes her head despondently. There has been no peeing at all.

11.02 p.m. – A strange noise echoes through the operating theatre. *Wiss wiss.* Is it the sound of a flow of urine splashing off the basin? *Wiss wissssss wissssss wiss wiss.* The sound appears to be man-made. *Wissssss wiiiiisssss* *shhhhh wisss wissss*. It's her mum. She appears to be making peeing sounds in the hope of encouraging Katrin. There is no pee-pee.

11.03 p.m. – *Wiisssss issss iisshhh wis wisssss*. The orthopaedic consultant hasn't a fucking clue what's going on as he glances over at me.

11.06 p.m. – Mum announces that she thinks Katrin is shy because of the people. I think Katrin is taking the piss out of us, as it were, and is just stalling.

11.08 p.m. – The 'wissing' is cut short as the exasperated nurse reaches in and yanks the basin out. There will be no more waiting for Katrin to pee. The orthopaedic consultant smiles at this no-nonsense attitude.

11.09 p.m. – Once more, I have my hand on the tray of drugs and approach Katrin. Her eyes flash at me and over to her mum. She pulls her in closer and whispers. 'She says she is ready to pee now!' I give a sideways, slightly condescending nod as I grab the cannula and rapidly send Katrin to sleep.

'She can pee when we're finished.'

275 – Perspectives

Although I understand what surgeons are trying to achieve with each operation, I'm pretty certain that it is probably harder than it looks. It's one thing looking at a few diagrams and reading the steps in the process, but actually applying the knowledge to a real scenario is quite different. We've all thrown a few wobblies trying to build an Ikea bed frame. There is a definite learning curve as you can see the stark contrast between the skills of a surgical SHO and those of a consultant surgeon. The consultant looks poised and slick (don't worry, the insults are coming), the SHO looks awkward and jittery. As anaesthetists, we get to witness all different types of surgery and I have a good idea of what is a hard operation and what is an easy one. I'd love to have a go at some of the easy ones. Easy: appendicectomy, grommets, removing a cyst. Hard: reconstructing a trachea, spinal fusion, reattaching a hand.

I'm not so sure that there is similar appreciation of complexity the other way around. Some surgeons are, of course, extremely conscientious and see the bigger picture. Others, not so much. The second group, I wager, see an unconscious body nicely positioned for the operation. It doesn't matter who put it there or how tricky it may have been to render the flesh-bag seemingly lifeless, provided it is ready and poised for surgery. They saunter in, complain about the positioning, and ask what took us so long before cracking the standard joke – 'Sure, you just have to put in the white stuff!'

This possible gulf in reciprocal understanding became apparent to me this morning. With eight cases on the list, it looked like a busy day, but the surgeon cheerfully announced that all the operations were relatively minor so we'd likely be finished early. I couldn't fault the argument that the cases were minor – they were. If there were eight limp flesh-bags all lined up in a row at the same time, we'd probably be finished in under two hours. The problem was that all the patients were ... problematic. From my perspective, this was one of the most challenging cohorts of patients I had been lucky enough to anaesthetise in the last nine months.

Patient 1 – Malignant hyperthermia risk, sleep apnoea, on home CPAP (continuous positive airway pressure) = *Could die.*

Patient 2 – Congenital myopathy. Severe mitral valve disease with evidence of heart failure = *Could end up in ICU. Or die.*

Patient 3 – Known difficult intubation, severe aortic stenosis = *Could die.*

Patient 4 – Syndrome I've never heard of = *I'll Google it up to see if they could die.*

Patient 5 – Syndrome I can't even pronounce = *See above.*

Patient 6 – Severe autistic spectrum disorder = *Could be traumatic.*

Patient 7 – Haemophilia = *Call the blood bank.*

Patient 8 – An ex-girlfriend's son = *I might die.*

As I scratched my head at where to begin, I gently suggested to the surgeon that it might take me some time to get my head around their problems and to anaesthetise them.

'Just give them some of the white stuff!' came the helpful reply.

276 – Wolf

I lost it in theatre today. I am ashamed to say I raised my voice. I shouted. I feel bad, but it got everyone's attention when I really needed it.

We had been operating on a premature baby with Down's syndrome. It was a big operation, but everything had gone well to this point. We had one last anaesthesia task to perform at the end of the operation. We had to switch the oral ETT to a nasal ETT, as it is easier to manage in PICU. This can be hazardous in tiny babies given the fact that their mouth and pharynx will have to accommodate two ETTs, a nasogastric tube (or two, in this case) and a set of forceps.

It was almost 3.30 p.m. I had taken no break for lunch, nor had any water since breakfast. I had woken up with a headache in the morning and it hadn't settled. I was happy the operation had gone well, but I couldn't wait to sit down and have something to eat and a cup of tea. The switching of the tubes (sounds like a biblical scene) was tricky and took longer than expected, but I was anxious that the tube not be dislodged accidentally, as I didn't particularly fancy having to replace it in a hurry. I was on high alert. Surprisingly, despite a baby being so small, the process of moving a sick one from the operating table into the tiny, ergonomically ridiculous incubators requires great skill and a degree in engineering. First and foremost, we have to protect the precious ETT. Secondly, we have to protect all the tiny cannulae and monitoring lines attached to the baby. Thirdly, we have to try to maintain the monitoring through-out the move. Anaesthetists get *very* anal about the move from one bed to the other. Our drip stand was holding six syringe-drivers, all in use, an epidural syringe-driver, intravenous fluids, two bags of intravenous feed (called 'total parenteral nutrition' or TPN for short) and another bag of fluids for the monitoring lines. This drip stand would also need to be manoeuvred around the incubator. Picture a baby suspended in a Christmas tree that, for some reason, needs to slow dance with a set of traffic lights.

We would have to move the baby down towards the end of the operating table, and remove the bottom section of the operating table before carefully inching the drip stand around in front of the baby and over to the other side, nearer the incubator. On my command, we started this process. Bit by bit, slowly but surely, all while protecting the precious tube and lines. The lines started to become taut, suggesting that the driver of the drip stand was not paying attention to what they were doing. They were at risk of moving the stand too far from the baby and pulling all the lines out. I looked up and realised that the driver was a student nurse doing the moving. I called everyone to stop, desperately trying to main-tain some slack in the lines. This was not the case for a student to be helping. I asked a more experienced nurse to take the wheel. We rescued the situation and thus we had completed the moving of the drip stand (biblical scene 2). Next, we removed the monitoring from the main monitor onto a portable transfer monitor as it would not reach across to the incubator when we moved the baby. The screen went dead. We now had no monitoring. *Deep breaths, Colin.*

It was far from ideal, but everything was rosy just before that moment, so I was happy to let the nursing staff it figure out. My head throbbed. My mouth was dry. After 60 seconds, which seemed like an hour, we had the monitoring back. All ok still.

Time for the moving of the infant (biblical scene 3). The big move was really only a move of about a metre from the operating table on my right to the incubator on my left. My registrar was in the 'receiving' position (no dirty jokes), ready to take the baby. A nurse stood by his side at the incubator. We checked everything was good before I disconnected the baby from the ventilator and moved her. Everything looked fine. I passed the ventilator tubing over the registrar to reconnect the baby to the ventilator. The tubing was pulled taut; it could barely reach. Someone had rolled the ventilator away from me during the move and now it was just a couple of inches too far away to reconnect. It was imperative to reconnect it before the oxygen levels started to drop. The receiving nurse yanked the tubing forcefully and connected it to the endotracheal tube. There is only one winner in the fight between a tiny baby and the heavy ventilator. As the nurse let go of the stretched tubing, it started to pull the ETT out of the child's nose. This was not good. If there was anything I did not want, it was for this tube to come out.

I looked at two things in rapid succession – firstly, the carbon dioxide trace. The only place carbon dioxide comes from in a ventilator circuit is exhaled by the patient when they breathe, so if it registers carbon dioxide, the ETT is in the right place. The ventilator showed a sliver of a carbon dioxide trace. The tube is most definitely on the way out. *God my head hurts*. Next, I glanced at the monitor to check the oxygen saturations. If the tube is not in place, then the oxygen levels will quickly drop. Someone had moved the portable monitor during the move and it was not in my eyeline. I couldn't see the number on the screen. *I'm so hungry*. Anaesthetists get remarkably tuned to the tone of the saturations monitor. The tone drops as the saturations drop. We use our ears when we can't use our eyes.

I announced quickly that I need to either get the baby closer to the ventilator or the ventilator needed to be closer to the baby to rescue the situation. Now all I could hear is noise. Loud noise. A constant din. A busy train station. There seemed to be chaos and the drone of a marching band in the operating theatre. I can't hear the saturations monitor. It's all I have. I can't hear anything. I'm thirsty. I'm irritable. I'm tired.

'QUIET! I can't hear the sats monitor!'

You could have heard a pin drop. Deathly silence. Peep, peep, peep goes the saturations monitor. My ears tell me it is ok, certainly over 90 per cent. Someone had repositioned the monitor for me to see. Yes, the saturations are 92 per cent. My registrar moved the baby closer to the ventilator and the tension on the little tube decreased. We saw a perfect carbon dioxide trace. There was no emergency, everything was ok.

Nobody said another word until we finished the move. The nurses didn't dare look me in the eye. I had never done this before. Once we had the baby settled and ready to go back to intensive care, I lifted my head and apologised for shouting. It is not in my nature. 'Hanger', it seems, is a real thing. The nurse manager replies with, 'Don't worry about it!' But I felt shitty.

I am not the first to raise their voice in an operating theatre and certainly will not be the last. There are tales of old where surgeons and anaesthetists would make nurses and registrars cry regularly. That type of behaviour wouldn't be acceptable today but we all regularly witness surgeons becoming irritable when the going gets tough in an operation. It can be stressful.

I recall a similar situation in London where we anaesthetised a child for a heart transplant at 3 a.m. Heart transplants are of great interest to many who rarely get to see them, so despite the time, the operating room was full of observers, nattering away in various corners of the room. In a similar scenario, the monitoring stopped working when the child was quite unstable. A calm gentleman of a consultant anaesthetist exploded with, 'Can everyone shut up? This isn't a fucking nightclub!'

281 – Scrub Trafficking

Scrubs: the uniform of the operating theatre. Standard issue, unflattering, oversized, multi-purpose, mystical coarse cotton pyjamas. No pressed shirt at home? Don't worry, you can put on scrubs. Cycling to work in the rain? Relax, you can put on some dry scrubs. You dropped some pesto out of your vegan sandwich onto your shirt? Just head to theatre and get some scrubs. Trying to hide an accidental pregnancy? Big baggy scrubs are your friends. Maybe you're just fat? Get a scrub size up. A child just pissed all over your leg? Clean scrubs will keep you right. Can't be arsed buying pyjamas for your home? Just steal some scrubs from work! It's Halloween and you have no costume? Pour some tomato ketchup all over the scrubs and use your imagination.

There's nothing worse than being forced to wear the wrong size of scrubs due to a lack of availability of your size. I don't know which is worse, too big or too small. Squeezing into a pair of small trousers is no mean feat. The fact that they're halfway up my shins is the least of my worries as any sudden movement is likely to have the arse split right up the middle. On the contrary, for me, wearing an XL top is like swimming in your dad's shirt that you were forced to wear to a family wedding as a skinny 12-year-old. The deep V-neck reveals far more chest hair than I'm comfortable with, never mind the possibility of a male nip-slip. Nobody wants to see that. Combine the XL top with the small bottoms and I might actually just prefer to wear a shirt and tie, the uniform of those doctors outside theatre, and join the never-ending clinic of a medical team.

Annoyingly, most hospitals have now made it relatively difficult for us to nick scrubs to bring home. Due to outrageous rates of scrubs going missing, most hospitals now employ a system where you have to check your scrubs in and out and maintain your 'credits'. No credits left, and you'll have to explain yourself. Fortunately, most of the children in the hospital would be capable of outsmarting the scrub machines, meaning we are all flush with credits. Although this system has reduced the number of sets of scrubs leaving the hospital, rogue scrubs often appear in every hospital.

Rogue scrubs, perhaps fed up with how they were being treated elsewhere, often turn up a long way from home. You see, whilst now all scrubs are generic, older sets of scrubs would be embossed with the hospital they belong to: Wexford General; Our Lady of Lourdes, Drogheda; or Santo Domingo Hospital, Port of Spain, Trinidad. I was reminded of this today as the nurse in charge was sporting a set of scrubs embossed with 'Mater Private'.[56] Now, this hospital is only across the city but later today I saw another pair with 'South Infirmary' clearly marked on them. That hospital is about 250 km away. *What the fuck is going on?* Maybe their home hospital used them too often or too little? Maybe their home hospital has a body-odour problem? Maybe I work with a bunch of thieves operating a national scrub-trafficking ring?

No. Scrubs go where they please, you can't control them.

282 – The Fast Show

Anaesthetists love to cancel cases, at least that's what the surgeons think. It's nothing to do with patient safety, it's just to annoy the surgeons. Ate a fry this morning? *That's a cancel.* Taking antibiotics for a chest infection? *That's a cancel.* You're having chest pain when you go out for a cigarette? *Cancel that.* You looked at the

---

56 They were actually embroidered, the fancy bastards.

anaesthetist the wrong way? *Who here can spell 'cancel'?* Your surgeon tells me you're a VIP? *Gimme a c … gimme an a …* You can only be operated on first because you're having your dog washed later? *You better believe that's a cancel.*

I'll let you all in on a secret. Realistically, we can anaesthetise anyone, at any time, in any condition and there's a 99.9 per cent chance that they will survive the operation. However, that does not, by any means, indicate that they will survive the remainder of their hospital stay unscathed and walk out the door. This is the crucial part to grasp. The hard part of surgery is the recovery and you need to be in optimal condition before embarking down that route. That is why anaesthetists may deem someone unfit for surgery. It doesn't mean it's cancelled forever, it just means we need to investigate that relentless chest pain before anything else. It is on these terms that we insist on fasting for any elective surgery. Us anaesthetists are risk averse, so why would we permit the unnecessary risk of you vomiting back up your eggs Benedict and landing in intensive care?

Back to the kids. If you think your wife/husband/sister/friend/neighbour suffers from hanger, then I dare you to walk into the surgical day ward in a children's hospital at 9 a.m. on any given weekday. The first children on the list are the lucky ones. They are into theatre by 8.30 a.m. and probably munching on breakfast, back in the day ward, by 10.30 a.m. We insist on six hours' fasting for food, and now one hour for clear fluids. Allowing kids to drink clear fluid (water, apple juice) up to an hour before anaesthesia goes some way to settling the hanger, but only slightly. Come 10 a.m. and little Alfie who normally devours his Coco-Pops at 5 a.m. is now literally throwing the toys out of the pram and screaming in the face of his desperate father. You glance over between the flailing arms and scrambling parents to see little Zoe who, in desperate times, is now attempting to eat some of the blocks of Lego in the play area. Steady on, Zoe, you're not due on the ENT list to retrieve a foreign body from your airway, you're here for an MRI scan.

Some of the starving children play the other card and go for the puppy eyes. A tear forms in the corner of Freddy's eye as he asks Dad, for the 345th time, if he can have some bread. Just some dry bread, Dad. Occasionally parents just relent. Fuck it. Here's your porridge, Emily. When asked why they didn't follow the fasting instructions they just sigh and tell us they couldn't take it any more. Emily was hungry. She beat me.

In theatre today, we sent for a patient at 11 a.m. A few minutes later, a toddler arrived at theatre reception with her father. As we flew through the first nursing checks, everything appeared to be in order: name, date of birth, hospital number ...

'Any allergies?'

'None.'

'Any regular medicines?'

'No.'

'Fasting since last night?'

'No.'

'Wait, what?'

'She had breakfast.'

'At what time?'

'8.30 a.m.'

'Why did you give her breakfast?'

'She was hungry!'

Sigh. Ok, I've seen it before. I can't imagine what it's like to starve your child. I've also learned that what constitutes a meal can differ between families. I'm hoping she only ate a grape. If this is the case, then I'd probably deem it safe to proceed. A plate of baked beans, hash browns and a sausage washed down with a Bloody Mary, maybe not.

'What did she eat?'

'A Twirl and a bag of crisps.'

What the actual fuck? This man has fed his toddler a chocolate bar and a bag of crisps for breakfast. I'm afraid I can't put her to sleep as it's only 3.5 hours since she's eaten. But obviously this is not the most remarkable thing about this interaction. For starters, she would usually have eaten herself to a great big 'cancel'. But things are different in a kids' hospital. We do recognise that people have taken time off work to get here. The kids are going nuts with the whole fasting thing, so we try to accommodate as much as possible. We did not cancel her operation, but sent her back to the day ward to wait until that silky milk chocolate and the stodgy remnants of her cheese and onion crisps had made their way through her stomach. In the meantime, we pointed Dad in the direction of the food pyramid and put in a call to the dietician.

283 – Close the Loop

Anaesthetists are involved in pretty much every emergency there is in a hospital. We manage things directly if they occur in theatre but often run to emergencies in every other part of the hospital – outpatients, the wards, intensive care, the emergency department, the corridor, the car park, a toilet, outside on the street, I've done all of them. The emergencies vary from things that are most definitely not emergencies to someone in a full cardiac arrest. Almost everyone who works in a hospital undergoes basic life-support (BLS) training and then some doctors and nurses undergo advanced cardiac life-support training (ACLS). There is also training for major trauma (ATLS) or for paediatric emergencies (APLS). So effectively, everyone who arrives at an emergency of any kind has some training. The courses teach a very methodical, step-wise approach to critical scenarios. They promote clear, direct communication with closed-loop interactions, meaning that we repeat the instruction to confirm that we have heard the instruction. There is always a team leader. If you ever watch a demonstration video of a terrible medical emergency, a cardiac arrest for example, the actors are all composed, speak directly to each other with purposeful statements, actions are carried out immediately and everything is very quiet and controlled.

This is a fantasy. This is like matching with a 24-year-old model on Tinder and skilfully securing a date in a trendy hip restaurant. When you arrive, you are actually in a chipper and meet a hairy 57-year-old man wearing a cocktail dress and vomit-stained stilettos. An emergency in the hospital is nothing like the videos. I mean, we manage to do what we need to do, eventually. However, the process of getting there involves a lot more noise, a lot more chaos, significant confusion and debris everywhere. You know it has been chaotic when you see packaging, empty syringes and various fluids strewn all over the floor. There is little closed loop communication and much more shouting into the ether. 'I NEED AN ET TUBE!' There are either none or multiple team leaders. 'WHO'S IN CHARGE HERE?' Several people are performing various different parts of the head-to-toe evaluation out of sync with each other. Not everyone is cool and collected, some are crying, some are freaking out. Accidents happen. The first ever cardiac arrest I attended I squirted a syringe full of adrenalin across the bed and into the eye of one of the cardiology nurses.

Chaos reigned today as the alarm bell went off in one of the theatres. I ran to assist one of my colleagues and the room quickly filled up with anaesthetists, nurses, cardiac surgeons, porters, the 1999 treble-winning Manchester United team, JFK and Red Rum. Trolley after trolley of extra equipment arrived. Resuscitation drugs, defibrillators, ultrasound machines, a bicycle pump, five litres of spiced rum, a Ouija board, a cement mixer and an Ordnance Survey map of the MacGillycuddy's Reeks. The room suddenly feels like the mosh pit at a Westlife concert – spine-tingling shrills, a dense din in the background and very claustrophobic.

I figured that we might need some advanced airway manoeuvres and infrequently used equipment. Commence the shouting into the ether. 'I need a double lumen ET tube, a bronchial blocker and a bronchoscope!' Who was I shouting to/at/for? I wish I knew, but lo and behold, after a brief interlude, some of the equipment arrived. But not all of it. I was missing a crucial bit of kit, like having a car but with a key that doesn't fit. I had not been specific enough with my ethereal request and only had myself to blame. Now we were losing a bit of time. I thought of those instruction videos where the communication is completely robotic, direct and with no added emotion. I saw one of our anaesthetic nurses – pupils dilated, ears pricked – seemingly awaiting instructions from whoever was next to shout the loudest. I pulled her quietly to the side and told her exactly what I needed and where to find it. Only moments later, I had all the kit ready to go, should we need it.

Ironically, and thankfully, we did not require any of the equipment I had been commanding faceless bodies to retrieve. I had been getting ahead of myself but, 'fail to prepare, prepare to fail'. Thanks, Dad. Despite years of working in intense and frankly scary emergencies, I finally understand why the American video robot doctors are so mechanistic. It's really the most efficient and controlled way to work in these scenarios. I say this, you say this back to me, we share a knowing glance and Bob's your uncle. I might start applying this 'closed loop' communication in my home life.

'Colin, refill my wine glass.'

'You wish for me to refill your wine glass, dear.'

'Yes.'

'Your wine glass has been refilled.'

285 – The Crying Game

You have to become accustomed to hearing children crying when you work in this environment. Walk anywhere in a children's hospital and you will hear multiple kids with the waterworks running. In the same way that my ears are tuned to differentiate between the different tones on the saturations monitor, I have become pretty good at recognising the different tunes of crying:

The hungry cry

Tone – low to mid-range

Additional sounds – occasional whining, possible screaming

Huff rate – infrequent

Associations – anaesthesia pending

Consolability – possible with suitable distraction, such as Peppa Pig or Paw Patrol

Location – frequently heard in the surgical day unit where fasting children may be spotted

Cure – food

The 'get me the fuck out of this place' cry

Tone – mid to high range

Additional sounds – audible rage at parents who promised they would be at the zoo

Huff rate – frequent, often uncontrollable

Associations – previous experience of hospitalisation

Consolability – difficult, may require heavy sedation

Location – hospital wide

Cure – getting the fuck out of the hospital

The painful cry

Tone – high range

Additional sounds – grunting, straining, grimacing

Huff rate – frequent

Associations – anaesthetist believing their regional block was working

Consolability – easy

Location – theatre recovery room, emergency department

Cure – a nice strong intravenous painkiller for the patient and an unwavering faith in their block for the anaesthetist

The 'I want my mummy' cry

Tone – low

Additional sounds – unique staccato of words intertwined with huffs

Huff rate – regular but possibly used for attention-seeking purposes

Associations – deserted by parents for painful surgery

Consolability – easy with presence of Mummy

Location – theatre recovery room

Cure – a nice strong intravenous painkiller. Or Mummy.

The delirious cry

Tone – low range

Additional sounds – moaning, speaking in tongues

Huff rate – none

Associations – staring into space, confusion, recent anaesthesia

Consolability – unpredictable, potential to lose their shit and advance to core meltdown

Location – theatre recovery room

Cure – a nice strong intravenous painkiller. Brave caregivers will ride the wave of the storm until the episode passes.

The fearful cry

Tone – high range

Additional sounds – shrieking, palpable fear

Huff rate – mandatory, purposeful

Associations – anxiety

Consolability – almost impossible
Location – hospital wide
Cure – time

While my ears and brain are able to tolerate most cries, probably because we can do something to relieve whatever the problem is, the fearful cry is a different beast. It is bone-chillingly awful. It gets to me every time. I have so much sympathy for the kids. The shrill is so mind-blowingly genuine that you would be forgiven for thinking the child was being tortured. In some ways, they may believe what is happening to them to be torture. We have to bear this in mind: children don't cry like that for no reason.

I was walking down the long corridor from theatre to the wards this afternoon when I started to hear the familiar sound. A scream. Another guttural scream. A pleading 'no, no, no'. A cry. A 'please, please, no'. A cry that became a dry retch and a fit of coughs. As I walked around the corner, I laid eyes on a young girl. She was skinny and pale with no hair on her head. Her mother carried her in her arms as she tried to force her way out of them. She was too weak to win the struggle. A nurse walked alongside with a wheelchair and pushing a drip stand. The child had a nasogastric tube in her nostril. Her lips were dry, cracked and blistered. The drip stand was supporting two syringe-drivers, one for fluids and another for the creamy liquid feed attached to the nasogastric tube. She had a visible Broviac line in her upper chest (a large, long, surgically implanted cannula for long-term use). The Broviac line was the dead giveaway, as you don't get yourself one of those unless you are very unwell and in for some long treatment. The child was clearly suffering the effects of chemotherapy – no hair, loss of weight, anaemia, mucositis, loss of appetite. I don't know what was terrifying her so much in the corridor, but she looked as if she was on a slow walk to some hellish place.

That sort of fearful cry is almost exclusively heard from kids who have a long-term illness who know only too well what may be coming around the corner. It is easy to forget sometimes that our patients are children and what is routine for an adult patient is terrifying for a child. Having a cannula placed is a piece of cake, unless it is the 100th time you have required one in your short time on Earth. The debilitating short-term effects of chemotherapy are easy to explain to an adult. Not so for a brave little girl.

289 – Up All Night

Practising medicine can be draining, both emotionally and physically. Over the years of training, I have felt like a functioning zombie at times. It is next to impossible to perform at 100 per cent at 5 a.m. when you have not yet been to bed. I can't recall any grave errors I have made at that time of the day, but I am sure I have made them. Sleep deprivation is a form of torture.

Almost all junior doctors now go home the morning after a night shift. It may be a 'night' in name only as it can be 16 or 24 hours in reality. Again, I have no figures to quantify how many errors may have been prevented when the walking dead are sent home in the morning, but it must be many. Standards of care are so much higher now that any medical error is unacceptable. But 'Well, he was up all night, so it's not surprising there was an error' should be more along the lines of 'Why was this doctor permitted to work such a long shift?' Ideally, shifts would be capped at 12 hours, but we are still a long way from that being universal, in Ireland anyway.

Trust is placed in talented registrars to manage most issues overnight. But consultants are always available over the phone and can be present in the hospital at short notice. The downside to that being that there is no mandatory 'post-call' day off for consultants. If you were in the hospital all night dealing with a very sick patient, there is no day off for you. This happens in almost all paediatric specialties, where consultant presence in the hospital in the early hours of the morning is normal. Anaesthesia is one of them.

I was in the hospital late last night, getting home to bed at approximately 3 a.m. But the alarm went at 6.30 a.m. and I was back up to face a full day in the operating theatre. You simply can't be tired. You have to focus. You must concentrate. Caffeine is your friend. Today's theatre list had changed late yesterday evening, but I had not been notified. We would now begin the day with a procedure on a very sick baby from the intensive care unit. Not what I wanted, given the palpable exhaustion I was experiencing. A stiff double espresso focused the mind, and before I knew it we were in theatre and I was feeling sharp.

The body is a phenomenal machine. The ability of our endogenous hormones to affect our mood, performance and focus is astounding. It is evolution for survival. You cannot sleep when being stalked by a lion. In this case, it was in fact survival we were dealing with. Not my own, but my patient's. That stirs the body into protective mode, as if it were your own child you were caring for. I feel no fatigue, no lapse in concentration. As soon as we safely return the baby to PICU, the adrenalin is gone and the exhaustion hits again. Another coffee and off we go again to protect the next vulnerable child.

I am lucky that our anaesthesia department operates like a family. We are a cohesive group. We are very aware of what went on in theatre overnight. We look after those colleagues who are working tired. Helping our colleagues, in reality, is designed to protect the patient from a good doctor making a bad error as a result of sleep deprivation. By early afternoon, another theatre had finished their operating list. The consultant anaesthetist covering that list came and permitted me to go home.

290 – The Unseen Workers

As day progresses to night in the hospital there is a change in shift. The nurses on the wards complete their long days. The night cleaners come in and scrub the high-traffic areas that can't be cleaned during the day. Security switch over and keep a close eye on the entrances and the ED overnight. I am on call and thus confined to theatre until all the work for the night is done. At about 10 p.m., as the surgeons are closing the skin on a long cardiac surgical operation that started in mid-afternoon, I decided it was time to have a cup of tea.

I lumber, a bit bleary-eyed, down the stairs and turn into the usually bustling tearoom. It is empty. The crockery has all been cleaned and put away, the chairs are stacked as if the floor has just been washed. Ordinarily, crockery is stacked, unwashed, in the sink. Our lack of dishwasher means the cleaning staff do most of the washing-up, despite signs pleading for people to clean up after themselves. I make myself a cup of tea and pull up a lonesome chair to catch up on some texts. The night cleaner walks in and I give him a nod. I don't know his name, but I spot his wiry frame arriving after 6 p.m. every day. He is quiet and moves about mostly unnoticed, keeping to himself.

As I finish my tea, I watch as he cleans the toaster and the battered Nespresso machine. Same thing, every night, with nobody around to notice who does the work. Not in any hurry, I stroll over to the sink and rinse out my mug before leaving it cleaned on the counter to dry. When I turn around, he is looking directly at me.

'You're the first person I have seen cleaning their mug this week,' he told me in an accent that I can't place.

'Really?'

'Yes. Everyone just leaves everything.'

I am no saint. My heart sank a little bit as I recall the many occasions that I have left my dirty dishes in the sink. The cleaners during the day seem to be continually washing plates. Occasionally, there is a legitimate reason for leaving things if one is in a hurry to get back to something ongoing in theatre, but most of us have no excuse. There are a lot of things we take for granted, working in a hospital. It takes hundreds, if not thousands, of staff to keep the place in good working order. Anaesthetists often complain (in jest) about never getting any thanks for doing their job, claiming surgeons get all the glory. Think about the guy who polishes the floors all night. Or the woman who tidies the changing rooms and cleans the toilets. Or the staff who work nights in the lab, alone, processing urgent blood results. They leave in the morning without being seen and you can be sure as shit that nobody says thanks to them.

292 – Robin Hood

I coolly slid out through the door and into the corridor, certain no one noticed what I had done. I had the contraband buried within my hands and now was rapidly cramming them into my scrub pocket. The PICU tearoom can be loud and busy mid-morning. It's easier to steal things when it's busy. There was too much action for anyone to notice me plunging my thieving hands into the fridge. If there were only two of us present, then my every move would have been seen. I would be left with no choice but to murder the witness, an option preferable to fessing up to the crime I had just committed.

I walked briskly from the PICU tearoom and out around the corner to find myself pushing through the double doors into theatre. I still had another 50 metres to get to my destination, but I still could feel the coldness of the bounty in my pocket. I pictured the scenes I would meet as I burst into the room, triumphant. A cheer, for sure. Hugs from the nursing staff, definitely. Maybe a parent would hear of my bravery and name their newborn child after me.

I tried to suppress a small grin, but I couldn't help it as I moved passed Theatre 7, then 6. As I reached the top of the staircase, I felt relief. I knew that when I skipped down the two flights to the theatre tearoom I would have gotten away with it. The perfect crime.

I marched into the tearoom with my head held high and my chest puffed out. I scanned the room to see three tables full of staff getting stuck into their breakfasts. Those with fruit and yoghurt looked delighted. Some had cereal; they too looked happy with their choice. But the majority looked miserable, dreary even. The thing they had in common? They were eating toast. Hot sliced pan was popping out of the industrial toaster at a rapid rate. The steaming, golden slices of toast singeing fingertips as they were directed onto plates. The beaming smiles would quickly turn to horror when they sat down. On face after face I saw desperation, disbelief, anger and then, ultimately, acceptance. They forced dry, matted pieces of toast into their mouths. The worst imaginable.

You see, there have been changes to our butter allocation this week. It has hit us hard. Some people have been said to stay at home sick rather than face this humiliation. Others say a nurse quit her job. The effects are filtering through the department. People are not happy. Every morning the plague of despair seems to consume another poor soul. You can't resurrect your day after a mouthful of dry toast. We used to get two full boxes of butter portions every day. Some say three back in the good old days. Now, we're down to one. When the box arrives, the vultures dive in and hoard those little envelopes of yellow heaven.

Not today, though. I had had enough. I couldn't just sit there and watch my colleagues descend into madness and the department into anarchy. As I flung the 30 pieces of carefully, individually wrapped butter onto the table, I could sense the mood change. I was no longer Colin Black, I was Robin Hood.

295 – Flipping the Bird

A premedicated young teenager with autism landed in the anaesthetic room. She arrived with her mother and, despite the early morning premedication cocktail, was quite visibly anxious. She reluctantly moved from the trolley over onto the operating table, all the while clutching her mother's right arm. Her eyes scanned the room, attempting to ascertain who was doing what.

No two kids with autism are the same. Yes, they have broad behavioural features that are common in order to receive a diagnosis, but the outward manifestations of these features can be quite different. This girl, I was told, was particularly distressed by being touched by anyone who was not one of her parents. But she was interactive, and certainly able to tell us this herself. Being placed under anaesthesia does require some degree of touch – after a premedication some kids need help to move onto the operating table, the nursing staff need to place some basic monitors on (e.g. the blood pressure cuff) and I need to either be allowed to hold a hand to site an IV cannula or place a mask over the face. I did my best to explain everything before we did it in an attempt to put her at ease. 'Is it ok if we check your identification badge?' 'Is it ok if we put the cuff on your arm?'

Probably the most important monitor we have is the saturation probe that loops around a finger. If I was going to get one monitor on her, it would be that one. I approached her with the small strip of Elastoplast that anchors the probe and told her that it was important for her to let me put it on one of her fingers.

'Anna, is it ok if I put this on one of your fingers?'

She shrugged – the premedication was having some effect.

'Is there any finger you'd prefer me to put it on?'

To my surprise, she replied with, 'How about this one?', before cocking her middle finger and lifting it up to face me. Was she flipping me the bird?! We all, mother included, looked at each other with some confusion. Our sideways glances all shared the same puzzlement – was she genuinely suggesting this was her preference, or was she telling me where to go? After some silence, as we wrapped the sats probe around this erect middle finger she piped up again.

'Can't any of you take a joke?'

303 – Chernobyl

It is a long walk down the theatre corridor for a toddler. From the reception to the furthermost theatre is about 60 metres. Sixty metres, at toddler pace, opens up a wide window for a full nuclear meltdown. There are many things that can trigger our little power plants into a core explosion, if the hunger and tiredness hasn't got them already. To make it from reception to any of our anaesthetic rooms you have to squeeze past equipment, walk past recovery and dart your way past many theatre staff. Someone looked at the toddler the wrong way? Meltdown. A child in recovery has a glass of lemonade? Meltdown. The realisation that you have been duped and are not on the way to the see the cows? Get the Geiger counter.

Our anaesthetic nurses collect parent and child from reception and guide them, skilfully, through the obstacle course to the destination of the anaesthetic room. Granted, we have ourselves many a meltdown in the anaesthetic room, but that is to be expected. Having one on the corridor, though? That's sooooo one-year-old. You're a big girl of four now, so no crying please. We tend to wheel out our patients, still anaesthetised, on a trolley to the recovery area where the recovery nursing staff wait for them to wake fully. There can be a lot of traffic and it's fairly common for a whizzing trolley to encounter a little wobbler insisting on doing the long walk from reception themselves. The sight of another child unconscious with an ETT or laryngeal mask sticking out of their gob is not one you wish to present to those arriving in theatre. But the anaesthetic nurses are masters of distraction. Our corridor is lined with pictures of cartoon animals and Disney characters. Before the child even notices a trolley coming, at the instruction of the anaesthetic nurse, they're in a parent's arms and we start the 'Who's that?' game.

There is a danger zone. A chicane. A bottleneck. At one single point, the corridor narrows and also meets the stairs from the changing rooms and tearoom. This means we have corridor traffic mixed with stair traffic. At this point, our cartoon wall gives way to a window into an unkempt and much less exciting courtyard. A courtyard with a pigeon problem. The pigeons don't give a shit. Actually, they give lots of shit. The courtyard is covered in pigeon shit. They are impossible to shift. A clever solution to keeping the actual pigeons (hard to stop the poo) out of the courtyard was to mount a net on the roof that covers the courtyard. Problem solved! No more unsavoury pigeons sitting on windowsills gawking into the theatre corridor. But they're still there, glaring down at us from the roof as we shimmy past each other in the bottleneck.

A number of weeks ago a dead pigeon appeared, suspended in the net over the courtyard. It was too far from any of the flat roofs to approach and pluck it out of the net. Hence, I have been watching this bird decay, slowly, over the last six weeks. The other pigeons continue to look at us, almost nudging each other in the ribs with delight over the situation. The ritual sacrifice of a fellow winged rat seems an intentional joke at our expense. It seems to leave them content, with an air of arrogance. Now that I know it's there, I can't help but glance out at it every time I walk past.

I spot my anaesthetic nurse accompanying our next patient down towards me, a coy-looking small boy, Tommy, holding her hand. As they approached the bottleneck, a colleague of mine whizzed past with a patient on the way to recovery. The anaesthetised patient always takes priority, so everyone stands aside to let them past. Our anaesthetic nurse lifted Tommy up out of the way. To prevent core meltdown, she turned a full 180 degrees and showed Tommy our uninspiring courtyard. Stuck for anything to point out, she prompted him to look up and see how sunny it was.

It was only when Tommy starting sobbing did she realise the problem here. Asides from Halloween perhaps, pointing out the rotting corpse of a flying rodent to a toddler would not be among our recommended distraction methods. The prospect of weeks of nightmares and a lifetime of ornithological trauma left Tommy with no option but to smash the big red meltdown button. Hoping for either a hole to open up in the floor or for a jet pack to burst him through the roof and out of theatre, he squirmed out of the nurse's arms and into his mum's. The nice quiet, gentle induction I had planned in the anaesthetic room has flown out the window with Tommy's soul, into the cooing pack of pigeons mocking me from the roof above.

307 – Mini-adventures

There are some particular days in work that are immensely satisfying. I'm proud to have worked so hard to get to this point. I feel privileged that surgeons and nurses trust me to do the tough cases with them. I'm honoured that parents put huge amounts of trust in me with their children. I'm lucky that I have this fantastic job. I feel this every day to some extent, but there are other days where this satisfaction submerges me. Those are the days when we are truly on the cutting edge of what is possible in medicine. Innovative surgery, critically ill children, rare diseases or really tiny babies.

It is the weekend and I am on call. We started with three really quite sick kids. A baby with a severe heart problem suffering from intractable fevers and very poor IV access needed a central line. A toddler had a huge abscess under her chin, pressing on her airway. Another toddler had a chest full of pus from a severe pneumonia that required a drain to be placed inside her chest. All of this was before we had to bring a baby to theatre for a bowel operation who wasn't even as heavy as a bag of sugar. The baby was about the weight of two iPhones (I just weighed mine). This is a truly tiny baby. For neonatologists, the paediatric doctors who look after neonates, though, this is probably quite big as they look after babies who may not even weigh 500 grams sometimes. All of these babies are *extremely* premature.

When I started studying medicine, a baby born before 26 weeks' gestation was thought to be too premature to survive and thus no care was offered. Over time, this target shifted to 25 weeks and then 24 weeks. Now, babies of less than 24 weeks' gestation can survive, given the right circumstances. It is not an easy journey; so many things can go wrong. Their tiny frames are not ready to be out in the world yet. They are cared for in the neonatal intensive care units (NICUs) which are located in maternity hospitals. Here, they are placed in incubators, protected and slowly fed. Their weight creeps up gram by gram. If a preemie requires surgery, they must be transferred to a paediatric hospital as it is not possible in the NICU or maternity hospital. A dangerous transfer for a baby this size. Tiny IV lines can be dislodged almost with a cough. Precarious ETTs can fall out if moved only half a centimetre.

One of the most common ailments requiring surgery in preemies is called necrotising enterocolitis (NEC). NEC occurs when the blood supply to the bowel is not sufficient to meet its metabolic demands. It can result in perforation of the bowel or even result in a section of bowel dying. In severe cases, it can be fatal. Our baby was in reasonable condition, all things considered. He had been born at 23 weeks and six days' gestation and was now nine days old (25 weeks and two days' 'corrected' gestation age). Our consultant general surgeon on call had accepted him for transfer and surgery. The plan was to bring a small piece of bowel out to the skin (a loop ileostomy, if you're interested) to give the diseased section of the bowel a chance to recuperate. Seems simple, but nothing is in a 650-gram shrimp. Although we do occasionally have babies this size in the paediatric hospital, it is not the norm and usually only temporary as they return to the NICU as soon as possible. It puts us all on edge, myself included. This would be the smallest baby I had ever managed alone.

You would assume it is easier to move a tiny baby compared to a 16-year-old. But it's quite the opposite. The process of moving a baby this size from the NICU to the PICU and then to theatre is a well-choreographed, but glacial, procession. Any abrupt movement and you can lose a precious piece of equipment. Our journey of 90 metres must have taken nearly 15 minutes as we inched our way to theatre. Moving from the incubator to the operating table takes just as much precision. It is such a tenuous faff that often, if the baby is extremely unwell, we will perform surgery in the intensive care unit lest we get into potentially fatal trouble whilst transporting the baby. Our journey was successful, and surgery commenced. The surgeons are only too aware that a long operation is not in the best interests of the baby at this age and they moved quickly. It was all done in half an hour.

During the operation, I had an unnerving moment when I realised that this baby, at 25 weeks and two days' gestational age, was the exact same age as my unborn child currently wriggling around inside my wife's uterus. I got a bit emotional at the thought, although I managed to hide it well (I think). It is cruel that our baby is still safe where it is supposed to be and this poor scrap is out here, prematurely fighting for survival. I sincerely hope this baby is doing well when ours is born in three months' time.

308 – Cluedo

When I arrive into work midweek, mine is frequently the first car in the car park. Over time, though, you start to notice some other early risers and what cars they drive. Leaving in the evenings, you get to know who owns all the other cars in the consultants' car

park. Spotting other people arriving early midweek is of no consequence to me as I know what planned operating list I am assigned
to on that day. But at the weekend, when I'm on call and still arriving early, the identity of the other early starters takes on a new
significance. I begin to wonder what's going on in the hospital.

Making small observations from the hospital car park, through
the corridor, into the changing rooms and up to theatre can inform
me of who is there and what might be happening in some corner of
the building. On the walk in, my mind will start making up scenarios of what lies ahead. The perfect weekend theatre day will involve
some straightforward operations in some healthy children. Maybe
an appendicectomy, maybe a simple broken bone or two and a few
lacerations that need fixing under anaesthesia. Nothing stressful.

If I spot the intensive care consultant's car in early at the weekend it tells me it's probably been a rough night in PICU. Were they
up managing medically unwell kids or is there a major trauma or a
small baby that needs surgery today? If I see the orthopaedic
surgeon's car early in the morning, I start to think the trauma list
might be huge and they are sorting the masses for surgery. Or
worse, they might be planning to revise a spinal fusion, which could
take all day. If I spot the general surgeon's car early in the morning,
I definitely start to get concerned that they are investigating a child
with a very worrisome abdomen either in ED or on the wards. The
worst car to see early in the morning at the weekend is that of the
cardiac surgeon or the cardiologist. Cardiac surgery is generally not
a weekend surgical specialty. There are few true cardiac surgery
emergencies that require immediate surgery and they are rare as
hen's teeth. If their car is spotted early at the weekend you can be
assured something serious is brewing which will most likely take
me all day to manage and, as a consequence, postponing all the
other emergencies until much later in the day.

This morning I saw one unidentified car (mixed feelings), parked
properly within the parking space (reassuring). On the walk in I

then glance through the window to see the entrance of the ED. How many ambulances are there? Are they all coming for surgery? Only one ambulance parked this morning. This could literally be anything, including an ambulance moving a patient *out* of the hospital, so it's best not to jump to conclusions. Next stop, the theatre tearoom. Today is Sunday and I had been on call overnight too, so I know that presently there is no ongoing surgery. But if I were to arrive early on Saturday morning (where a different consultant anaesthetist was on overnight) and find no nurses arriving for their shift, it is reasonable to assume they are performing some major operation that could just not wait. Are there half-finished cups of tea? Are they still warm? This morning there was no sign of life. They're either already working or not yet here.

I stroll into the changing rooms after I scan the tearoom. Is there a locker flung open and not closed as if someone was running to theatre? Who own the shoes that looked like they were kicked off in a hurry? *Hang on a second, I can see the perfusionist's shoes there.* The perfusionist is the person who not only runs the cardio-pulmonary bypass machine in cardiac surgery but who also prepares the ECMO circuits used to support the sickest children we care for. My mind races over scenarios – is there an ongoing cardiac arrest and they are asking for ECMO support? Is one of the cardiac surgery post-op kids deteriorating and needing ECMO? Does the presence of these shoes indicate I am about to have a horrific day in work?

Most of the terrible scenarios I have flashing in front of me are false. I could drive myself insane if I only thought about what *might* happen later in the day or draw conclusions from entirely innocuous 'clues'. But you can't ever stop thinking about it just a little. Anaesthetists are primed, trained and ready to work in stressful and dire situations. This doesn't mean that I necessarily *look forward* to them all the time. If it needs to be done, it needs to be done, but I don't think that I, or any of my colleagues, wish for a constant stream of critical emergencies. Especially not at the weekend. The same speculative thoughts are the ones that consume you a little bit as you try and close your eyes for sleep when you're on call. The sleep is never quite as restful.

After I got changed today, I sprung up the stairs to theatre to see what lay ahead. Deathly silence. There was no emergency surgery. I popped to PICU. There was no ECMO. I looked at the emergency list – there were a few minor trauma cases listed for the day. I went back downstairs to the tearoom. Now a few nurses greeted me as they sat down with their tea. The perfusionist must have just left his shoes behind.

310 – From the Sublime to the Ridiculous

An annual tradition on the run-up to Christmas is 'Ho Ho Ho Day', which happens to be today. All staff are invited to dress up in whatever costumes they desire, festive or otherwise. We are limited in what we can wear in theatre, but there are a few painted faces. Out of theatre, though, it's fair game. Multiple Santas patrol the halls. There are reindeer, elves and snowmen going about their clinical duties. I'm not sure who loves it more, the kids or the staff. I bump into one of the radiology consultants who discusses a case with me, dressed head to toe like Will Ferrell's character in *Elf*. It's impossible not to smile.

With this sort of dress-up comes a degree of absurdity. While it is not recommended to be in costume when breaking bad news to a family, if you have a straightforward day planned then it is encouraged to join in. I feel somewhat self-conscious as I explain the risks of anaesthesia wearing a snowman-covered scrub cap that both parents and child seem fixated on. The day got a little bit more ridiculous in the afternoon. As I walked down a quiet corridor, a consultant surgeon peered around the corner. 'You're exactly who I'm looking for!' The surgeon grabbed my arm and pulled me into another corridor, gesturing at a man-sized patient being wheeled into a side room on a trolley.

'He's one of the staff. He felt like he was about to pass out and had to lie down on the floor. We helped him onto a trolley. He's definitely got atrial fibrillation. I could feel it!' the surgeon announced triumphantly.

Atrial fibrillation ('a fib') is the most common arrhythmia found in adults but is almost non-existent in kids. Where the heart rhythm usually arises in an area called the sinoatrial (SA) node in the right atrium, with atrial fibrillation it arises elsewhere, resulting in a very distinct staccato rhythm that can be easily felt in the pulse. It can leave people experiencing palpitations and occasionally feeling faint. It can be managed with drugs, an electrical shock (cardioversion) or a catheter ablation procedure. As if the day couldn't become even more ridiculous, I thought, a surgeon is diagnosing arrhythmias.

I wandered into the side room where one of the nurses (wearing a reindeer hat) had wheeled the staff member. Sure enough, he confirmed that he suffered from atrial fibrillation. *They don't make surgeons like they used to.* But his pulse felt normal to me. You can flip back to a normal rhythm just as easily as you flip out of it. Seeing as he still felt like shit, I summoned a cardiac technician to come and obtain an ECG to look at his heart rhythm more closely. Moments later, in burst a panting elf pushing the ECG machine in the door, his long curly elf shoes almost causing him to trip on the end of the trolley. After an ECG was quickly performed, we could see that the atrial fibrillation had returned.

Managing this would be a piece of cake in an adult hospital, but, completely unsure as to what I was and was not allowed to do to an adult in a children's hospital, I thought it better to ask some advice on whether he needed to attend an adult hospital. I left him with an elf, a reindeer and a (festive?) Catwoman as I ran off to find a cardiologist. I located one, wearing an awful Christmas jumper with built-in light show, and shoved a few ECGs under his nose. With his advice in tow I marched back down to the elf protector and my oversized patient.

I was, apparently, forbidden from administering any IV drugs to an adult patient. I obeyed the advice, seeing as I'd prefer to keep my job, and told our staff member that we better get him to an adult hospital if the a.fib doesn't resolve. Accepting this, we turned to leave the side room only to find the Grinch standing in the doorway. 'I've heard you've been a bad boy, causing trouble all day.'

312 – Death

In medicine, we are taught the value of empathy. We are taught to listen intently. We are taught to be the advocate for the patient. We are taught to communicate. We are taught to be honest. We are taught to be all those things and more, but yet remain detached. We are taught not to become emotionally invested in our patients. To do so would be exhausting, distressing and a rapid road to burnout and personal distress. We are taught to do all those things but also to manage the expectations of patients and their families. Present the facts and allow them to process and make informed choices. Estimate risk, give percentages, give an opinion if asked. But it is not advisable to make decisions based on our own emotions. Our decisions must be evidence based and rational. But it is simply impossible not to feel invested in a patient. It is natural to be rooting for them and hoping that they overcome whatever obstacles they face. It is human to feel like this.

I wasn't due to be in work today, but I had to follow up on a baby on whom we performed emergency surgery yesterday. The baby had suffered a prolonged cardiac arrest 24 hours before, a long way from our hospital. They had been completely healthy and thriving up to that point. The baby and parents had arrived in our hospital, many hours later, fighting for their life. There was truly an imminent risk of death, with only slim chance of the child surviving the necessary surgery, but we had to try. Overnight I had been thinking about nothing else. I didn't sleep well. I had to come in to see the baby for myself.

As I walked up the stairs, I feared the worst. The sliver of hope that the baby might survive drained from me when I walked through the doors of the PICU. The intensive care team were disconnecting the monitors and removing some of the many drips. I saw the parents being slowly ushered into the corner of the room into a seat. I watched as the PICU consultant removed the ETT from the baby's nose before handing the infant over to their parents. I watched as the curtain was drawn around them. I could see nothing more, but I could hear the crying, gently at first but then without restraint. I witnessed the expressions on the faces of the PICU staff, bravely stoic but with more than a hint of sorrow in each of their eyes. I promptly left the PICU and headed for my car.

I have never cried in the hospital, but fought the tears back many times. I am always aware of my emotions but rarely express exactly how I am feeling, and certainly not in a work environment. I have been known to become overwhelmed with emotion, as anyone who was at our wedding can attest to as I huffed and blubbed my way through my vows. As I sat in my car, it was one of those moments. I had a brief but cleansing outburst of tears. I don't know exactly what it was about this child that affected me. I have witnessed many adults and children die in the intensive care unit. I think it is the thought of our baby, yet to be born, that has me choking up. Our baby is expected to be healthy, but so was this baby. Not only that, but this baby had been thriving. Less than 24 hours later, the lives of the parents have changed forever. I picture myself in their shoes. I am overcome with love for our own baby whom I am yet to even meet.

313 – The Hulk

'Jesus Christ, he's an animal!'

We were being overpowered by an infant called Theo. All hands on deck, get reinforcements! He was a mere 10 kilograms in weight and I had just anaesthetised him for a pretty major operation. So major, in fact, that I had requested a post-operative bed in PICU for him. The surgery had gone very well so I had decided I would extubate him in the operating theatre before transferring him to PICU. He was full of strong painkillers and sedatives, so I expected him to wake up slowly and gently. He might cough a little bit as we removed his ETT, but I imagined he would fall into a natural sleep fairly quickly thereafter. I knew the intensive care nurse would thank me for sending over a calm, awake, pain-free, quiet toddler. She was sure to have a quiet night looking after him.

We awaited Theo's emergence from anaesthesia. He was breathing well but not yet stirring so I took the opportunity to suction out the back of his throat to remove any saliva that may have pooled there when he was asleep. He didn't budge. *We've a bit of time before this chap wakes up.* As I chatted to the nurses, 10 minutes passed and Theo appeared to still be deep in the land of nod. But soon, he started to cough and grimace. This is usually the first thing people do when they come out of their anaesthetic coma. The awareness of the ETT in their trachea leads them to cough, at which point we can safely remove it knowing that the presence of the cough means the patient can protect their own airway.

Theo began to roll over to his right-hand side and I pulled the tube out. He let out another cough, then a growl. 'Ggrreeuughhhhh!' I prepared for the impending cry that most kids let out as soon as they wake up. But no, it was another growl. 'Aaaaaarrggghh!' At this point he had managed to fully roll over onto his belly, eyes still closed. This was not the ideal position to be in considering I was keen to give him some oxygen and he also had two large surgical drains emerging from his chest. But soon, Theo had hoisted himself onto all fours. Eyes closed, growling like a lion and now facing me head on. The two nurses and I attempted to roll him back onto his back. But he wouldn't budge. He knelt there, statuesque. He growled again. 'Eeeeeemmmgghhh!' *He can't be, can he?* He's going for it. This little beast is trying to stand up.

He forced his way into a downward facing dog position, arse in the air, all his floppy hair dangling above the mattress. A nurse steadied his hips. We tried to get him to lie down again but he pushed us away. *Fucking hell, we better just let him do what he wants here.* He let out another roar. 'Gggrrrrreeeaaaahhhh!' He was now on his feet, eyes still closed, seemingly semi-conscious. A nurse steadied him so he wouldn't fall over. His left hand reached up to his face and he yanked his nasogastric tube clean out of his nose. 'Raaaaaaaaaagh!' The same hand went to his right wrist and, with a swift yank, out came the line I had placed in his radial artery. A jet of blood sprayed his clean, white sheets. A third nurse had now appeared and immediately put pressure on his wrist.

Fearing for our own lives at this stage, I made the decision to give him some extra pain relief and some sedation to get him under control. It did nothing. He stood there, eyes closed, refusing to lie down with two hosepipe-sized drains in his chest. I expected his skin to soon turn green.

At this point he turned to face the nurse who had been steadying him from behind. He raised his arms up towards her neck and went in for the hug. She duly obliged. He now stood there, deep in embrace, with his head buried into her shoulder. She gently lifted him up and out of the cot and sat down. Soon the growls turned to heavy breathing and Theo was asleep again. He just wanted a hug. A few minutes later, with him sound asleep, we attempted the big move to place him back in his cot. The instant the reassuring pressure of the embrace waned, he opened his eyes and started crying. The instant the embrace was reinstated, he went back to sleep.

'There's only one thing for it. You're going to have to hug him all the way back to the PICU.'

We started the walk over to the PICU with an empty cot, being trailed by our nurse and Theo. Another nurse followed, holding his drains, like a bridesmaid with the bride's train. The PICU is used to sick kids, most of whom are heavily sedated in their beds with no prospect of jumping out into the arms of a passer-by. I visibly saw the hearts melting as the PICU nursing staff watched our nurse carry him to the far corner of the unit. We sent for his parents to come over immediately. Theo the Hulk spent the entire night sleeping in his mother's arms in a chair, with little to no interest in retiring to his cot.

316 – Grandmaster Rash

Ask most doctors what specialty they know the least about, and I'd wager that one of the most popular replies would be dermatology. Except of course if you are a dermatologist. Although sometimes I don't really believe that the dermatologists know what they are looking at when presented with a rash. The skin is a bit of a mystery to me. Where I can remember being taught at least some morsel of information about every other organ in the body in medical school, I struggle to think of anyone ever presenting us with some easily digestible nuggets of knowledge about rashes. I say rashes because why else would you need to see the dermatologist? It's always a rash. I later learned that a good treatment regimen for rashes is that if it is wet then keep it dry and if it is dry then keep it wet. And put some steroids on it.[57] Anaesthetists know nothing about rashes.

I received a call today from a surgical SHO to inform me that a baby had come in for pre-assessment for surgery which was scheduled to take place in two days' time. I was due to be the anaesthetist

---

57 This is not medical advice.

that day and the baby had a strange rash on their arm. I reminded the SHO that I am an anaesthetist and do not have the requisite skill set to differentiate eczema from measles from leprosy from Ebola. Nevertheless, I was summoned to review the child as the SHO had promised the parents that the consultant anaesthetist – Rash Wizard, Grandmaster Rash, the Rashmeister General – would soon be on the way. Practising my diagnosing face on the way up the stairs, I wondered what type of rash I might be faced with. Would it be the red one, the large red one, lots of little red ones, the scaly one, the bumpy red one, the sort of purply one, the one that is gone by the time I get there, or the one that is just dried-in ketchup.

As I introduced myself to the parents, who appeared delighted that I was about to shed some light on the genesis of this dermatological puzzle, I spotted a bright and bouncing baby boy. The fact that he looked well was a good thing; this probably wasn't a serious rash. Mum rolled up the leg of his trousers to reveal the troublesome area. I got down on my knees for a closer look. I squinted my eyes to appear like my brain was dusting off some old dermatology notes to come to the diagnosis on the spot. It appeared as if we were dealing with a reddish-purply one that was a bit hard. Not something I had ever come across before. We all agreed that it looked weird.

'What do you think it is?'

I haven't a fucking clue, but it's definitely not ketchup.

'I'm not sure, to be honest. Rashes aren't my strong point.'

The surgical SHO, appearing somewhat disappointed that she had summoned an equally inept 'dermatologist' to consult, suggested we ask the actual dermatologists to see the child. Great idea! Everyone was happy with the plan, except the dermatologist on the phone who eventually allowed us to send the baby down to their busy outpatient clinic to have a look. The SHO promised to call me when they had a diagnosis.

A couple of hours later, my phone rang.

'Dr Black, it's the surgical SHO. The baby has been seen by the dermatologist.'

'Great, thank you. What did they say?'

'They didn't know what it was. They just prescribed some steroid cream.'

317 – Shame

If you assume that doctors and nurses are healthy just because they understand healthcare then you'd be wrong. One just has to have a stroll through the wards, intensive care or theatre and investigate what lies in each of the tearooms. Many patients leave treats for staff around Christmas, but they very quickly pile up. And you'd be out of your mind to think that any of that is *not* going to be consumed in a gluttonous Christmas orgy. I guarantee it will be hoovered up in mere minutes like the festive piranhas that we are. On any given day you will find stacks of mince pies, assorted cakes, cheese boards and, of course, the dreaded tin of Cadbury's Roses.

I have eaten so many Roses at this stage that the sight of them makes my stomach start to churn. Every time. That said, my average Christmas Roses intake stands at about 15,423 sweets. They used to have a monopoly, but Celebrations and Mini Heroes now also appear in prominent positions strewn across wards nation-wide. Some poor people appear to be ashamed of their addiction to these little doses of dopamine. As I walked into the male changing rooms today, I spotted a wrapper on the floor. On close inspection it was that of a blue Rose. I breezed past on my way to the toilet when I spotted another on the floor beside the sink. A pink one. I opened the door of the cubicle to spot four more Roses wrappers ditched by the side of the toilet bowl. An assortment of colours at this point. Is it so bad to want to eat Roses all day long? Do you think people will judge if your gorge the whole tin yourself? Do you enjoy sitting on the toilet with food going in one end and coming out …? It's ok to be addicted. Half the battle is admitting you have a problem. Please talk to someone, I'm sure you're not alone.

It must be tough to feel you have to eat your Christmas treats in the toilet but, my God, man, have some self-control. After a detour to the tearoom, I plodded up the stairs with a mince pie, a slice of lemon drizzle cake and a mouthful of cookies crumbling down the front of my scrubs.

318 – Comfort

What is unique about a children's hospital is that often you are not only treating the patient, but one or two parents also. In an adult hospital, doctors are under no obligation to share any information about a patient's condition with family members unless they are explicitly permitted to do so by the patient themselves. The information regarding your health as an adult is for you and you only, no matter how insistent a family member may be; if you don't want to share a diagnosis or openly discuss treatment, that is up to you, the patient.[58]

Paediatric practice is different for obvious reasons. It's difficult to explain the concept of a cardiopulmonary bypass machine to a toddler who is watching the same episode of *Blue's Clues* for the 34th time. They're just not *that* interested, for some reason. Children can sign their own consent forms when they hit 16 years of age, though.[59] But for younger kids, the parents are the main

---

58 There are some exceptions to this – a person who cannot understand the information they are receiving (e.g. dementia, severe learning disability, in a coma, for example). In these circumstances it is the norm to discuss care with the next of kin.

59 They can do so even earlier if they are deemed to be 'Gillick competent' (i.e. they can understand the pros and cons of receiving a treatment).

GAS MAN

gatekeeper for clinical decisions. That's not to say parents of those over 16 are not involved in making decisions, it's just that the child is given more autonomy. Relinquishing some control to the teenager can bring some relief to parents who are stressed about the decision-making process. We often forget this fact as we are so focused on the child. Putting the child at ease is of course our primary concern, but we should never forget the fact that parents are vulnerable too. Who knows what kind of other home/work/life stressors they have? The sight of their unwell child may tip them over the edge.

That is why there are many supports for parents in children's hospitals. They range from parental accommodation to help with transport and food if necessary. There are staff dedicated to helping parents cope with the burden of their child being in hospital, sometimes for weeks. But there are often completely unsung heroes that help parents through difficult times. When we are anaesthetising a child in theatre, we usually permit a parent to join us. Often, it is the parents who don't want to leave the kid, even if the kid is totally chilled about the whole process. As the child falls asleep, the parent is whisked out of the room. We don't, in that moment, have the luxury of time to empathise and support the parents. They are permitted a quick kiss and a wave before being shown the door.[60]

This is where our unsung heroes shine. Our healthcare assistants (HCAs), who in theatre are responsible for keeping stock up to date, cleaning between cases and the like, escort the parents out of the theatre department. They are the first point of contact when a parent has entrusted a stranger with their child. Parents may sometimes feel like they have abandoned their child. Your natural instinct is to be with your child at all times. In fact, parents frequently ask

---

60 A colleague in London, struggling to communicate with a parent with poor English, once gestured to his cheek, suggesting Dad could kiss the child before leaving, only to end up with a sloppy, moustachioed puck from the dad on his own cheek.

to stay for the surgery or wait in the corridor outside the theatre. The best I can say to them is, 'This is going to take three hours. Go and have some lunch and try to relax.' *Relax?* What a cop-out. Of course they won't relax. That is why it's so important that the first point of contact recognises how the parents are reacting to the separation event and says the right thing. Our HCAs are almost professional psychologists. It's a true skill.

Today, a parent completely broke down in the anaesthetic room as their child fell asleep. The mother, in floods of tears, collapsed over the top of the child, covering their chest and abdomen and making it very difficult for me to keep the mask over the child's face. It was getting dangerous. The child had suffered a bad burn a few days prior. I believed the mother felt responsible for the accident. It was only when her child was unconscious, and not able to hear her, that her true feelings about the incident came to the fore. It is in these situations that a skilled HCA recognises both that I need to do my job and that the parent is very vulnerable. Our HCA managed to pry the woman away from her son and gently led her to the door as she sobbed. I could just see through the crack in the door as our HCA uttered some inaudible words before the mother threw her arms around her.

331 – BAO

I often cringe when I look at the letters attached to my name as part of my medical degree – MB BCh BAO. MB: *Medicinae Baccalaureus* (Bachelor of Medicine) – fine. BCh – *Baccalaureus Chirurgiae* (Bachelor of Surgery) – fine. BAO: *Baccalaureus in Arte Obstetricia* (Bachelor in the Art of Obstetrics) – I'm sorry, what? I'm a Bachelor in the *Art* of Obstetrics. Have you ever heard anything so wanky in your entire life? The declaration that one's field is beyond science and reason and has crossed over into the world of art reeks of self-aggrandisement. Can anyone spell 'delusions of grandeur?'[61] Now although I was just the epidural monkey, I did actually work in a maternity hospital once upon a time. I've worked hard to see the comparisons, but there wasn't much in the way of fanciful artistry when observing an obstetrician locking a suction cup to a baby's head, leaning their full weight into it and pulling so hard that one would be forgiven for thinking the aim of childbirth was to pull the baby's head clean off the torso. Paint *that*, Dalí.

It's not just obstetricians who fancy themselves as artists. As a student and a junior doctor, I frequently heard it from ageing physicians too. The declaration would usually come from an old school physician catastrophising that 'the art of clinical examination' is being lost on us young doctors. 'Too reliant on investigations, you lot are!' There followed a tiresome lecture on the time they diagnosed ulcerative colitis only from hearing the diarrhoea hit the toilet bowl or the time they tasted the pus from a wound in order to select the appropriate antibiotic.

'Young man, describe the murmur of mitral stenosis.'

'I don't need to, I'll just get an echo if I hear a murmur.'

'The art is sadly waning!'

What's wrong with just being a doctor?![62] Is that not enough? Was your mind set on art school but pressure from Dr Dad forced you into a career in medicine? What's wrong with getting scans? Surely it makes everything easier and more reliable. Anyone? *Anyone?* Art is creating something new from nothing. Art gives us a new perspective on something mundane. Art is taking independent materials and fashioning something amazing. I don't get any of

---

61 Before any obstetricians get angry, I will point out that it is far from the current batch of excellent obstetricians that decided the degree should include the word 'art'; this is a relic of ancient times. Do some of them still think they're artists? No comment.

62 The irony of writing a book is not lost on me.

that from listening for the sound of shit rumbling through some poor sod's bowels.

There is, of course, an obvious place in medicine to play the art card: surgery. A plastic surgeon who literally creates a new ear from cartilage harvested from elsewhere on the body – that is art to me. The cardiac surgeon who uses perspective and depth perception to re-route blood at the perfect angle deep within the chambers of a heart – that is art. Until today, I never really appreciated the art of the brutes. Those banging, sawing, clattering, wrenching, drilling, screwing meathead orthopaedic surgeons. On any ordinary day, the sounds from the orthopaedic theatre would be best suited to a construction site, minus the hard hats but including the cement (yes, they use bone cement). Surely there is no delicacy to that?

The skeleton has been artfully depicted since the days of anatomists like Leonardo da Vinci to painters like Van Gogh and Cézanne and many more. It is a beautiful thing to see exposed in surgery, probably because the bones are palpable just beneath the surface of our skin. I watched, in awe, again today as the orthopaedic surgeon performed a posterior spinal fusion to correct the spine of a teenager with scoliosis.

The surgeon exposes the entire length of the spine, from neck to pelvis, through one long incision. The bones become apparent as they peel away the large stabilising spinal muscles. It is a wondrous sight to see the spinous processes aligned, like the bony prominences one would associate with a dinosaur. It amazes me every time I see it, although today I have really observed with great interest. Sometimes, as anaesthetists, buried in our notes, we can miss the nuances of the work happening on the other side of the drapes.

Correction of this long, severe and disfiguring curvature of scoliosis is art. I watch as he moves with intent, purposefully and confidently selecting the angle for each screw to bore down into the vertebrae. He gently turns the screw to the desired depth – not enough and the metalwork will be unstable, too far and the screw can enter the spinal cord. Slowly, over the course of six hours, this contorted, primordial skeleton evolves to a metal-laden, bionic man of the future. The twists and rotations of the spine are ever more evident when the angles at which the bolts and screws emerge from the bone below are appreciated.

The operation builds to the crescendo, the final brush stroke. The long metal rods are gently moulded with heavy pliers to the desired shape of the new spine. The rods are gradually eased onto the screws lining the edges of the spine, like trees on a winding avenue. With each tightening manoeuvre the spine slowly edges into its new position, inching closer to the straight spine that was until now forever moving in the wrong direction. The job is done.

BAO – Bachelor in the Art of Orthopaedics.

334 – Decisions

The list is busy. It's almost 2 p.m. and I haven't stopped yet for breakfast, let alone lunch. I see a window approaching. A healthy child is up next in between seemingly endless hordes of complex children. I start the case with my registrar and bolt out the front door of theatre, ravenous. I have already missed whatever the canteen was offering up so I head for the coffee shop. A hefty queue awaits me. I'll just have to wait, my stomach growling like a bear, threatening to wake a baby sleeping in a bassinet beside the queue.

As the queue slowly moves, I begin salivating at the prospect of my lunch. There are only two customers ahead of me now, a porter who has ordered a pre-prepared sandwich and a mother with her son, who I guess is about six. We inch closer; mother and son are up. She is clear and to the point: 'I'd like a plain wrap with some mayonnaise, chicken and tomatoes.' *Not bad, I suppose. I think you need a bit of cheese if you were to ask me. And the sun-dried tomatoes are better.* Her son is up next. 'White bread!' he exclaims. *Good man, we're on the way.* 'Butter!' *He's going for it.* There follows a moment of uncertainty. His eyes scan the generous deli and all the possible combinations. I'm no mathematician but there must be several billion possibilities; it can be hard sometimes to craft the perfect sandwich. He looks at the cheeses – cheddar, mozzarella, feta and goats' cheese. 'Mum, do I like those?' After his near-flawless start, he is flagging. Maybe if I move my stomach a bit closer to the back of his head he might take the churning as a cue to hurry up.

'You like that one,' as his mother gestures towards the cheddar. Safe. Now is not the time to be experimenting with feta. She turns to me with a smile and mouths a 'sorry' in my direction. 'Not a problem,' I reply, also wondering which section of the deli to fall into should I collapse of starvation. 'What else?' asks the counter staff. His eyes scan again. He takes a step left towards the rainbow of condiments and starts pointing.

'What's that one?' he asks the staff.

'Mayonnaise.'

'And that one?'

'Garlic mayonnaise.'

'And that one?'

'Taco sauce.'

Mum intervenes, 'What are you looking for?'

'Ketchup.'

'Can you put some ketchup on it for him.'

Has my hunger just turned to nausea? He had made a good start but we're at the point of no return now with his butter, cheddar cheese and ketchup selections. *I think some hot chicken might turn this around.* I turn around to see the queue now out the door with a few heads bobbing out of line in an attempt to figure out the hold-up. The sandwich prince now takes three steps to the right, drawn to the hot section. *He's going to save it, a chicken fillet.* But no, he walks past the chicken fillets to the rest of the hot food. Here you have the remnants of breakfast, a chicken curry, a quiche and some boiled rice. He stands fixated here, his little cogs whirring. Twenty seconds pass. Thirty. Mum is feeling the squeeze from the queue behind.

'Come on, pick something else,' she urges.

He extends his index finger, like ET phoning home his final selection.

'I want that!'

'That's rice.'

'Yes.'

'Are you sure?'

'Yes.'

Mum, turning to the staff, 'Can you put a bit of rice in it for him, please.' She turns to me and shrugs her shoulders as if I, a paediatric doctor, should understand this selection. *Don't look at me, I only put them asleep. I don't know what's wrong with your odd son and his freaky sandwich.* The boy stands, hands out, in great anticipation, as the sandwich is delivered to him on a paper plate. He gazes at it in awe, admiring the fine choice he has just made. I turn to the staff, coldly and desperately barking my regimented order, somewhat jealous of the wonder in the eyes of the little weirdo with his cheese, ketchup and boiled rice sandwich.

337 – A-poo-calypse Now

Disfiguring and extremely painful, bad burns don't heal quickly, and in some ways you never fully recover, sporting the scars for the rest of your life. While burns are a tragic affliction for any patient, it carries extra poignancy when it is a child. 'Their whole life ahead of them' is the phrase that actually rings true in these situations. I won't bore you with the classification of burns, but in children the vast majority are as a result of boiling water scalds. Fire, chemical or electrical burns can occur, but I can count on one hand how many times I've seen a case of those. The piping hot cup of tea, the boiling pot on the hob or even a bathtub that is just far too warm. Even picturing all the potential household hazards has me racked with fear over the toddler who will be cruising around my home in a year's time.

Not all burns require a trip to theatre. Some require specialist dressings and follow-up, although in saying this some very distressed kids need to come to theatre for things as seemingly innocuous as a dressing change. Others require the full monty: multiple skin grafts, dressing changes and a long stay in hospital. Our plastic surgeons are excellent. The skin grafts and other procedures they perform can have fantastic cosmetic results. Unfortunately for the kids, some of these surgeries are awfully painful.

In cases of extensive, full-thickness burns, the patient can be incredibly sick. The melting away of normal skin leaves the body incapable of holding onto moisture, and thus the victims can become severely dehydrated. Multi-organ failure due to burns is not unheard of. The other side to having all these exposed wounds is the threat of infection via the weeping sores. Though their dressings do need to be changed, this is not done daily as it is just too bloody sore. This results in some of the dressings becoming quite 'fragrant' over the course of a few days. On top of this, patients with widespread burns drop their temperature very quickly, so we have to be hyper-aware of this fact and keep the temperature in the operating theatre at the level where you'd be more comfortable in the nip. But we realise that it's probably frowned upon, so we all just sweat.

I anaesthetised a toddler today. She had been in intensive care briefly, following a bad burn, but was on the mend. She was coming to theatre today for a dressing change and possibly another skin graft. As soon as she arrived in theatre, you could smell the wounds. The soft granulation tissue was doing its best to heal but, at this stage, was most definitely colonised with some bacteria. It was particularly pungent, though, almost like a toilet that hadn't been cleaned in a few weeks. After she had been anaesthetised, I set about trying to find a decent site to insert a new long-term IV line. She had lost many cannulas over the preceding weeks so it was time for something longer term. I figured I would try for the femoral vein in the groin, seeing as it was somewhat remote from the burns on her neck, chest and arms. She had pulled a pot of boiling water onto herself.

With this aroma of congealed human flesh and a room temperature more suitable to a Middle Eastern desert hospital with no air-conditioning, I was already sweating. The smell was particularly notable today. I had never smelled a burn like this. Which bacteria could possibly produce a smell as prickly as this? I removed her nappy to expose the groin and get to work. *Whhoooooooshhh.* Like an airborne ton of shitty bricks, it hit me. I gagged. In her nappy lay one of the most catastrophic shits man has ever witnessed. Acidic and tangy, the smell engulfed me. It was everywhere. It was no burn we had been smelling today, it had been this rancid nappy.

I glanced around; there were only two other nurses in the room and they had been doing paperwork in the corner. There was no way they witnessed my horrific discovery. I had the chance to turn back the clock. *Could I do this? Of course I could.* I closed the nappy back over and went to start writing some of my own notes. When a few more nurses were in tow, I looked over my shoulder and nonchalantly made the request, 'Would someone mind exposing her groin – I need to put in a new line.' I went back to my notes until I heard the gasps.

'What is it?' I exclaimed, feigning surprise.

'This is disgusting!' came the reply. 'I'll have to clean this before you go anywhere near her.'

'You sure? Thanks.'

Yes, I am a bad, bad man. I ignored that poo and left it for someone with more guts than me to sort out. It's like putting an empty milk carton back into the fridge. If the milk carton was made of shit. Am I sorry? A bit. Would I do it again? In a heartbeat.

343 – Max Power

'There are three ways to do things: the right way,
the wrong way and the Max Power way!'
'Isn't the Max Power way the wrong way?'
'Yeah, but faster!'

– The Simpsons

There are two classic ways to perform an inhalational induction in children:

The right way – a calm and cooperative child permits you, or their parent, to gently hold the mask over their nose and mouth while they are distracted with toys, funny faces, age-appropriate jokes, bubbles and puppies. Neither child nor parent suffers any stress and everyone lives happily ever after.

The wrong way – a distressed child, tormented at the idea of even being in the hospital, spits out every premedication in an act of defiance and refuses to enter the theatre department. They cling to their parent and cry inconsolably as they are carried into the anaesthetic room. They scream at the sight of anyone in blue scrubs and aggressively bat away the mask. They bury their head in their parent's chest, dig their nails in and bite at any exposed piece of flesh. Multiple people overpower the child, claiming they don't understand, before the mask is forcefully clamped over their nose and mouth and they eventually fall asleep in floods of tears.

Today I learned the 'Max Power' way to perform an inhalational induction. A young boy and his mother arrived in the operating theatre. He looked coy, she looked fed up with waiting. He tried to sit up on her knee, but she picked him up and plonked him directly onto the operating table. Admiring her gumption, we performed the anaesthetic 'time-out', our final check before we begin. During this, the boy begins to sob. 'I don't want to go to sleep.' Mum ignores his whimpering. She explains that he is the youngest of her five kids, all of whom have had an anaesthetic at some stage. She's been here before, she knows the score. She's from inner-city Dublin and her no-nonsense attitude is evident.

I grab the mask and show it to the lad. He's not particularly impressed with either the mask or my banter. He pushes me away and facing Mum he crosses his arms, tears on his face, and declares, 'I'm not doing it!' We have to be very careful about any physical restraint of a child. In an ideal world we'd never have to do it, but kids are independent creatures and evidently don't always appreciate what we're doing. If some sort of restraint looks on the cards, I always wait until the parent suggests it and document it, just to avoid any situations where parents reflect on what has happened and post-event decide they weren't happy with how the situation was handled.

I looked at the mother, but she was glaring at her son. 'You're doing it. We talked about this.' I move forward to have another go, but he has made his mind up about me. Mum reaches over to me, grabs the mask out of my hand and, facing the boy, plonks it directly onto his face. Ordinarily, we use one hand for the mask and place another hand on the back of the child's head to maintain mask contact, but also to support their head when they start to get sleepy. All technique was out the window now, as she just pressed forward and to my surprise, the boy stayed sitting upright and pressed his nose back against her, almost defiantly. With his face inside the mask, his protests continued.

'I don't want to do it!'

'All your bleedin' brothers did it and they're grand.'

'... huff ... huff.'

'We'll get a McDonald's after, ok?'

'... huff ... ok.'

'Now just keep breathing the stuff in.'

Now she shot a glance over at me as if to say, 'Jack up the gas there, doc.' Daring not to disagree, I did what I was told and cranked it to the max. Max Power on the gas. Full steam ahead. Seconds later, the little guy got wobbly and we caught his head and lowered him to the table. Mum sprung up, 'Allright, there yis go,' and made for the exit. Get that woman a job.

348 – Old-fashioned

'I have important friends,' replied our healthcare assistant.

It was late in the afternoon, at the weekend. We had slowly plodded our way through some emergency cases in the morning and we were set to have a break for lunch. Due to my generalised laziness around preparation for weekend work, I had once again neglected to bring any lunch with me. This was knowing full well that the food options were limited at the weekend. There was no canteen open, only a coffee shop with a limited number of options compared to a weekday. Despite this, I was looking forward to my sandwich with my stomach rampantly gurgling suggesting the 'intermittent fasting' regimen I have been trying was more gastronomically challenging than expected. My phone rings. The general surgical consultant. There is a baby with a very worrying-looking abdomen in the PICU. Surgery is required, fast. There would be no lunch for us.

I am often amazed at how we, as medical professionals, neglect our own well-being. Lack of sleep, dehydration, skipping meals, not exercising or, more worryingly, using alcohol as a coping mechanism for stress. While a laparotomy in a small baby is stressful, you'll be glad to hear I didn't prepare with an Old Fashioned. But I didn't take even ten minutes to eat a sandwich or drink some water. I just pressed on, as I have always done. I would always delay my gratification. Finish all the work, and *then* have a break. Study for 14 hours and *then* eat your dinner. Don't celebrate exams until they're *all* completed (even if the finish line was three years down the road). The constant demand for a doctor's (or nurse's) attention in a hospital is unrelenting. This has eased somewhat, as a consultant, because the registrars deal with many of the minor distractions.

Physician burnout is becoming much more of a recognised phenomenon. Overworked junior doctors are not helped by having some of their, frankly, insane rosters ratified by the powers that be. I recall being at a professional development seminar as a trainee where a man who worked nine to five, Monday to Friday, lectured us on the importance of eight hours' sleep per night. Half of the attendees (including myself) were attending having not slept the night before following a 24-hour shift in the hospital. He did not spot the irony. Such is the demand for tasks being completed immediately, junior doctors neglect their own well-being to tend to the patients' needs. The interruptions never stop. A plastic surgery SHO was scrubbed in theatre recently and I witnessed his pager alarm 12 times in a 30-minute operation. He told me he had received 145 pages the day before. No wonder people don't have time to drink some water.

A cynic might reply to these 'complaints' by stating that this is the path we chose. They are right. Old or retired consultants might reply by saying that they've all worked in these conditions. They are right. Management might tell us that we are here to help the patients first and foremost. They are right. They are all right, but those attitudes are outdated and old-fashioned. They miss the point. Demands on services are greater than they have ever been before. Everyone is stressed: doctors, nurses, patients, managers. But none of us are any use to patients burnt out.[63] My willingness to skip some basic human needs in the blink of an eyelid is a symptom of this being accepted practice in a hospital. I am the consultant

---

63 I'd like to stress that I, personally, am not at the burnt-out stage.

anaesthetist now, so I can delay the start of the next operation for 15 minutes to ensure the staff are fed and watered. But I sometimes don't even apply this basic standard to myself.

We worked through lunch and into the late afternoon to help the baby as best we could. The operation went well. I had forgotten my hunger until we had finished the surgery, the adrenaline keeping it at bay. But as soon as we had returned the baby to PICU, the gurgling resumed like waves crashing against the sea front. I headed to the theatre tearoom to see if I could muster some toast, only to find trays of vegetables, chips, crispy chicken and spring rolls. Surely a mirage – my eyes are deceiving me. The theatre nurses were tucking in, as were the porters and healthcare assistants.

'Where did the food come from?' I asked.

The kitchen staff, only there at the weekend to feed the patients, knowing we were working hard on a tiny human, had fixed us some food at the request of our healthcare assistant.

351 – Manners

Around the hospital, there are templates for communication to aid staff nurses to communicate specific, crucial information to doctors on the other end of the phone in the form of the ISBAR tool.[64] This *aide-mémoire* is stuck on the walls near phones all over the hospital and has been proven to be successful, particularly in empowering younger nursing staff to vocalise concerns to doctors.

There are other reminders that are slightly more questionable in terms of their target audience and function. Today I came across a

---

64 ISBAR: I = Identification (who you are, where you are, what patient are we talking about), S = situation (what is the problem that has prompted the call), B = Background (a brief synopsis of the patient's background), A = Assessment/Action (what do you think is wrong, what have you done so far), R = Requirement (what do you want from the person you are calling).

sticker plastered over a phone receiver. On initial inspection, one would be forgiven for thinking this was a toy phone that had been removed from a four-year-old's Montessori classroom. It was literally instructions on how to answer the phone and speak. The instructions were as follows:

ANSWERING THE PHONE:
Hello
Location
Name
Grade
How can I help you?

These basic instructions are only missing a diagram indicating where to place the phone receiver. *No, not on your testicles, Tony!* I'm not sure why the first letter of each word was highlighted, either – 'HLNGH' is not an acronym that rolls off the tongue. Is this the stage we've got to where grown adults need to be told to say 'hello' when they pick up the phone? I would love to know the standard of call that prompted management to insist that this sticker was necessary for our Neanderthal staff. '*What the fuck do you want, shithead?*'

Frighteningly, this is not even close to the range of other instructional signage that I have come across in hospitals. My favourite one was in a male changing room where a sign had been placed over the sinks saying: 'The sinks are for washing hands only. Please do not wash your feet in the sink.' A female friend of mine raised the bar when she informed me of a sign in another hospital: 'Please do not defecate in the shower.' In the *female* changing rooms. I don't know why I find this more bizarre in a female changing room – as if this would actually be quite common and acceptable amongst the men.

361 – We Like to Party

When you are preparing for a medical interview, there are a few stock scenarios that you must prepare for, as you will likely be asked one of them. They are usually related to human factors, workplace bullying, drug abuse or that sort of thing. They go along the lines of:

> Your consultant has turned up to work smelling of alcohol – what would you do?
> You have caught your consultant stealing fentanyl – what would you do?
> Your consultant is racially abusing a healthcare assistant – what would you do?
> Your consultant is being sexually inappropriate to a colleague – what would you do?
> You spot a packet of white powder in your consultant's locker – what would you do?
> Your consultant listens exclusively to One Direction – how would you murder him?
> Your consultant is seen Botoxing his face – how would you ask him to give some to you?
> Your consultant parks her sports car in the disabled spaces – which key would you use to damage her car?

Now aside from thinking what sort of maniac/party animal your consultant is (it's always the consultant), you are expected to demonstrate the need to prioritise patient safety, act with discretion, gather information, be non-confrontational, be supportive and escalate appropriately (free tips there for anyone doing interviews). We prepare a template for tackling these issues without ever expecting to have to put them into action, but I did today.

Now before anyone gets concerned, nobody was drinking/taking drugs/stealing/being abusive or anything of the sort. A staff member approached me to discuss how another staff member was treating them. It caught me off guard, as I do not know the staff member particularly well, but at the same time I felt privileged and humbled that they chose me to talk to. My 'resting bitchy face' clearly still demonstrates some level of approachability.[65] I talked to both parties, a resolution was reached and, personally, I felt a little bit more consultant-y.

Now I just need to get on with consuming vast quantities of cocaine in my Maserati while being more sexually and racially inappropriate to the staff, and I could be *that* legend of a consultant in the interview scenarios.

364 – Never a Dull Moment

It was late afternoon; things seemed to be quiet in the department. The usually bustling recovery was almost empty. There were no CNMs marching up and down the corridor. My own list had finished. I took the opportunity to nip to the office and reply to a few emails. Twenty minutes later, I nonchalantly strolled back to the theatre office on my way to heading home. I peered in the door to see if any souls were around for a chat. Empty. I peered into recovery. Empty. I casually plonked myself into a seat to review the operating lists for the following day.

A moment later, I heard the unmistakable patter of running feet. I glanced and saw a blurry silhouette of a porter running out of theatre. Then I saw the distinct silhouette of a cardiac surgery registrar sprinting in the other direction, back into theatre. A sprinting heart surgeon is never a reassuring sight. I got up to investigate. I walked down the theatre corridor, and all appeared empty, even the

---

65 Note to self: look more bitchy to avoid awkward conversations.

cardiac surgery theatre itself. The last theatre on the long walk is the cardiac cath lab. I heard some stirring. Then some shouting. Then some monitoring alarms. I increased my pace into a jog and pushed open the door of the control room. Through the large viewing window, I saw 15 or 20 people in the throes of managing a cardiac arrest.

There were three consultant anaesthetists and two registrars performing CPR. Two cardiac surgery registrars were scrubbed and another watching. An experienced theatre nurse was preparing an operating trolley. Two consultant cardiologists were standing back and talking animatedly. Nurses were running in every direction grabbing equipment. The porter who passed the office in a hurry burst through the doors carrying several bags of blood. Then, just as I suspected, two perfusionists wheeled in the ECMO circuit. It became apparent that a baby with a severe cardiac problem had suffered a cardiac arrest just after a life-saving procedure in the cath lab. The only way to a place of safety would appear to be ECMO (extracorporeal membrane oxygenation), which replaces the function of the arrested heart like cardiopulmonary bypass.

The cardiac surgeons had the unenviable job of trying to open the neck of the baby to access the tiny jugular vein and carotid artery. They would then need to gently thread two enormous cannulae into the vessels and place them in perfect position, while minimising blood loss. All this must be done on a moving target, as the vigorous chest compressions from ongoing CPR would preclude any stillness. ECMO in this scenario is called extra-corporeal life support (ECLS). It is very rare and is only really possible if a patient suffers a cardiac arrest inside, or very near, a hospital where this is possible. There are only two hospitals with this capability in Ireland. So, in some twisted way, the baby was lucky that this occurred in theatre.

I made myself available to help in any way. In these situations, we always take direction from the team who were present when the emergency began, as they know the patient best. I took ownership of making adjustments to the ventilator and directing a registrar to make notes and time all the ongoing events. A small but critical role. The team worked like a well-oiled machine. We paused, just momentarily, as the surgeons slid the second cannula into place and connected the tubing for the ECMO circuit. One final, but crucial, check for air bubbles before the perfusionist called 'Going on ECMO!', to the relief of the rest of the team.

The team stopped CPR as the ECMO machine whizzed into action. We glanced at the monitor – 35 minutes. Thirty-five minutes from the start of the cardiac arrest to crashing onto ECMO. To put that into perspective, that involves putting out the alarm, starting CPR, gathering the specific ECMO team, retrieving the equipment, setting up the equipment, continuing effective CPR, painting and draping the patient and performing extremely delicate surgery. Not bad. Moments after the restoration of some effective blood flow on ECMO, the heart rhythm appeared to be normal again. However, the baby was still gravely unwell – 35 minutes of CPR was still 35 minutes of CPR. The infant's heart would likely take days or even weeks to recover. There would also be a chance that it may never recover. Prognosticating at this stage is pointless. The next few days will be critical.

All in a day's work.

365 – The Exit Exam

What? No fireworks? No plaque for the wall? No guard of honour? No early retirement? Today is just another day for the hospital but it marks my first anniversary as a consultant. It is most certainly a milestone, but a personal one only, as no one else is even aware that they're now officially stuck with me as a colleague for the next 30 years. It marks the end of the standard one-year probationary period, and I am well and truly locked in for the long haul. The head of our department informed me that he had signed off on my probation already last week. I am now free to start slashing tyres in the car park, turning up late for work and stealing expensive medical equipment because I officially have a job for life. *Plain sailing for life boys – time to put my expensive loafers up onto that mahogany desk in my corner office.*

It was almost as if today's case was set up as an overwhelmingly complex exit exam for consultancy. It is apparently completely by coincidence that the most challenging case I have worked on all year is listed for today, my one-year anniversary. *Blow out the candles and get into theatre.* It is a proper test. This case had been flagged on my radar last week, but it was only over the weekend that the penny dropped on the coincidental scheduling. But here I am, ready to embark on a mammoth operation in what feels like make or break time for determining if I have matured over the course of the year.

Our patient today is a baby girl who has been stuck in PICU, on a ventilator, since birth. She has multiple complex medical and surgical issues. She has major abdominal, vascular, lung, airway and cardiac problems, placing any intervention in the highest risk category. A haircut might be problematic. The poor kid has already been on ECMO for a period of time and had several other high-risk procedures in theatre. The other trips to theatre have ranged from being entirely abandoned, to stomach-churning 'snatch-and-grab' operations, to some moderately successful, but temporary, solutions. But she is no closer to escaping the intensive care unit.

She is a favourite amongst the PICU staff. It is impossible not to be rooting for a patient who has, in reality, grown up in the intensive care unit. From tiny baby to now being a fairly chunky one with a personality. At first glance, this little girl appears to be strong and robust, but it is likely she will have a slow demise to a premature death if we sit on our hands. There are innumerable consultants involved in her care across all specialties – cardiology, cardiac surgery, general surgery, respiratory, neonatology, infectious diseases, ENT surgery, intensive care and anaesthesia. As it should be, there have been many multi-disciplinary team meetings to discuss the best course of action to give her the best chance of survival. There is only one thing for it: a high-risk surgical procedure. There can be no more waiting.

Kids are really quite robust; they can bounce back from what appears to be certain death to walking out of the hospital a couple of weeks later. In contrast to adult intensive care, PICU has fewer long-term patients but we still have some, like this little girl, who spend weeks or even months stuck in the same cubicle. That puts children at risk of all the complications of intensive care – infections, repeated painful procedures, loss of muscle mass, weight loss, arrested development and the long-term effects of sedative medications.

Over the last week I have been to PICU to visit this girl several times and to take direction from the PICU doctors who have been looking after her. Their input is invaluable to me as they have been caring for her directly over many months. But being intimately involved in the minutiae of a patient's care can be suffocating. It can be refreshing to arrive at the bedside of a long-stay patient and take a broader, wide-angled look at the overall picture. It has been the best way for me to prepare for the case. This approach has allowed me to not ruminate and make things complicated. As I am only borrowing her for a few crucial hours, I decide to focus on the major issues and ignore some of the minor details that the PICU team work hard to manage on a daily basis.

Due to the gravity of the case, we have an unprecedented number of consultants in theatre. I am the lead anaesthetist, but there is another consultant anaesthetist available. There are five consultant surgeons directly involved in the case, with two operating at any one time. Over the course of the day, three more consultant anaesthetists and two intensivists drop in to see how things are progressing, such is the interest in her operation. Everyone is rooting for her.

In any high-risk operation, we must prepare for the worst, while hoping for the best. Being prepared for the worst enables us to manage our own expectations about the surgery. If X happens, we will do Y. I am expecting problems with A, so to counteract that I will do B. Any anxiety or fear in the operating theatre is as a result of the unknown. We can prepare thoroughly for the 'known unknowns'. Through multi-disciplinary meetings and endless investigations, we can arm ourselves with the tools we will need to make quick and rational decisions. But like anything else, it's the 'unknown unknowns' that are most terrifying. These are rare and we must trust our training to shine a light down those dark tunnels if we fall foul of one.

This little girl flew through the operation, much to everyone's surprise. It was a well-prepared, dedicated, invested and empathic team of doctors, surgeons, nurses, pharmacists, physios, porters, healthcare assistants and, hell, even anaesthetists. She almost got a cheer as she returned to PICU this afternoon, such was the delight of all the staff. But like most other complicated cases, this successful operation is just another stepping-stone on her path to recovery. She is far from cured, and faces many more months of life in the hospital.

EPILOGUE

As I completed the final draft of this book, I stroked my beard and gave myself a large pat on the back as I saved what was the complete manuscript. *Well done, Colin.* It was finally finished. Then I deleted the entire epilogue. Then I thought I should continue the diary entries. Then I thought I would have to write a completely different book, given the new circumstances I was working in.

Covid 19 had arrived in Ireland. In the early stages, we battened down the hatches in work. I taught other staff to correctly don and 'doff' (I'm reasonably sure this word was invented for this pandemic) personal protective equipment. We cancelled elective operating lists and made contingency plans for a mass outbreak. Although the disease does not seem to affect kids in the same way as adults, the fear was that they were asymptomatic harbingers of the virus, ready to infect any unsuspecting adult. We bickered about how we would manage an anaesthetic of an infected child, or even an infection-free child. We half expected to get moved to work in adult hospitals. We waited for the surge in cases that would overwhelm our health service. As we sat in the deathly quiet hospital, Covid-19 was a lot closer than I could have imagined.

Four days before her due date, my wife became unwell at home. She lay on the sofa, pretending nothing was wrong and began to rigor.[66] I took her temperature: 38.5 Celsius. A fever. What else could it be? Less than 36 hours later, my wife was one of the first 300 people in Ireland to test positive for Covid-19, and the first pregnant woman. Before you reach for the Kleenex, do not fear, the story has a happy ending. In the same 36 hours, she delivered a healthy baby girl. Her body, in the midst of fever, decided enough was enough, and she went into spontaneous labour. Despite being sick, she insisted on experiencing labour the way she wanted, with minimal medical intervention and no pain relief. My wife dominated both the virus and labour itself. After six hours of labour, we had our daughter. The awe I have for my wife increased tenfold. Wonder Woman. It was not all that we imagined, though, considering healthcare workers in space suits don't regularly feature in maternity units. But we have our own unique story to tell our grandchildren in 50 years' time.

My wife recovered extremely well from the virus and we took our baby home after just ten hours in hospital. Luckily, our daughter is perfect. I am not a religious man, but it is a miracle. I was shocked to witness what they call a 'term' baby with 'average' weight not requiring immediate intubation and life-changing surgery. Who knew they even existed? My outlook on what constitutes a healthy baby is so very warped from working with the sickest and most unfortunate children in the country. It's like living inside *The Truman Show* bubble, not bearing witness to all the joy a healthy child brings outside the hospital. I have garnered a whole new respect and admiration for the parents who blow away any adversity put in their path and adjust their lives to the needs of their sick children. They are amazing people.

From our perch, at the top of the operating table, anaesthetists can observe everything. We register thousands of data points during a

---

66 'Rigoring' is the uncontrollable, involuntary shaking you get in the throes of, or lead-up to, a fever.

day of clinical work in a busy operating list. Heart rate, temperature, blood pressure, saturations, airway pressures, carbon dioxide, flows, vapour, percentages, drugs, dosages, millilitres, sizes, shapes, patterns, cues, triggers. It's not sufficient to merely notice an anomaly, but what it means in the broader context of the clinical situation. There is a complex triangle of connections between the anaesthetist, surgeon and patient. All the observations are connected in some way, shape or form and can be manipulated by any point of the triangle.

But it is impossible not to observe the connections between people too. The operating department, intensive care and the hospital throng with people. There are many sides to this bustling hive. Parents pace the corridor with worry or beam when they are reunited with their child after surgery. Children run to the fish tank with joy, or joylessly vomit on the floor. Porters ferry patients around the hospital singing or philosophising. Cleaning staff meander through the corridors with quiet intent. Nurses ready medications with focus or giggle with the kids. Doctors scribble illegibly in notes or make treatment plans with clarity. It is busy, it is thriving, it is a marketplace. People and patients interact with each other in more ways than they can imagine. They influence each other's moods, they shape each other's experience, they remain in each other's memories. Our hospital experiences are entirely dependent on the interactions we have with other people.

The yearning for connection is even more evident from here, in the middle of a healthcare crisis. We work, but it is not the same. We talk, but from a distance. We express ourselves, but from behind a mask. We're brave, but we are scared. We feel we are surviving, but not living. The connections are there, but they don't feel the same. They are lined with a subtext of anxiety and fear. It is evident in how our eyes meet, or how we greet each other. I miss the craic. I miss normal work. I miss the stuff I don't even like. But it will pass, and we will be a better healthcare team on the other side, of that I am certain.

ACKNOWLEDGEMENTS

This book would not have been possible without the inadvertent help of all the patients and their families that I am lucky enough to care for on a daily basis. It is a joy to work with every child that I am responsible for, and rest assured any future patients who think I'm writing notes on them, I've stopped paying attention. (That's a joke, in case my legal editor is rolling up their sleeves.) I would also like to acknowledge all my colleagues – porters, cleaners, health-care assistants, managers, secretaries, security men, the women in the coffee shop, the guy whose name I don't know who keeps nodding at me, radiographers, nurses and, of course, other doctors. Again, this book would not have been possible without all of these people, and let's be honest: you're going to have to pretend you enjoyed this book as I've another 30 years until I retire. So, you can all practise your fake smiles. *It was great, Colin.* Special thanks to Dr Barry Lyons whose advice on all things ethical, medico-legal and football related were most welcome.

I would also like to say thanks to Eabhann, my wonderwoman of a wife and harshest critic. 'You sound like a dick, Colin,' was the best advice I got when writing this book. The little chicken, Laoise, didn't exist in the outside world when I was writing this but sure look, you can show this to your pals in school and tell them you're famous. My own parents, Thomas and Helen, my sister Amy and my in-laws, Ger and Edel, were all early readers of the first drafts.

I thank them for putting their time into reading those rough pages and confirming my own suspicions that *Gas Man* was brilliant.

I'd like to give special thanks to Tom Chapman, my brother-in-law, who guided me through the maze of a literary contract and was a tremendous help.

Thanks go to my editorial team at HarperCollins. Conor Nagle, who convinced me to sign a contract with them after demonstrating excitement for the book akin to a 6-year-old on Christmas morning. Nora Mahony, my editor, for being a good sport and spelling out all the numbers I wrote. 4; 6; 7; 22; 309; 4,532; 19,234; 2,139,824 – are you going to type all those out before we publish? Notable thanks also to Catherine Gough, Patricia McVeigh and Joel Simons.

GLOSSARY

Medicine can be a complicated world of acronyms and shorthand. It's hard to keep up; use this as a reference.

ABG – arterial blood gas
CICU – cardiac intensive care unit
CPB – cardiopulmonary bypass
CPR – cardiopulmonary resuscitation
CT – computed tomography
ECG – electrocardiogram
ECMO – extra-corporeal membrane oxygenation
ED – emergency department
ETT – endotracheal tube
GA – general anaesthesia/anaesthetic
GP – general practitioner
ICU – intensive care unit
IV – intravenous
LMA – laryngeal mask airway
MRI – magnetic resonance imaging
NICU – neonatal intensive care unit
PICU – paediatric intensive care unit
SHO – senior house officer
SpR – specialist registrar